# CARIBBEAN HERBALISM

## Traditional Wisdom and Modern Herbal Healing

Aleya Fraser

Text copyright © 2025 Aleya Fraser. Design and concept copyright © 2025 Ulysses Press and its licensors. All rights reserved. Any unauthorized duplication in whole or in part or dissemination of this edition by any means (including but not limited to photocopying, electronic devices, digital versions, and the internet) will be prosecuted to the fullest extent of the law.

Published by:
Ulysses Press
an imprint of The Stable Book Group
32 Court Street, Suite 2109
Brooklyn, NY 11201
www.ulyssespress.com

ISBN: 978-1-64604-816-8
Library of Congress Control Number: 2025930779

Printed in the United States
10  9  8  7  6  5  4  3  2  1

Acquisitions editor: Kierra Sondereker
Managing editor: Claire Chun
Editor: Pat Harris
Proofreader: Sherian Brown
Production: Abbey Gregory, Yesenia Garcia-Lopez
Cover design and artwork: Catherine McElvane
Interior artwork: All from shutterstock.com. Chapter start and folio hibiscus © Caraulan Art; p. 6 © Peter Hermes Furian; pp. 29, 32, 35, 43, 50, 55, 57, 59, 70, 72, 74, 80, 82, 89, 91, 95, 96, 98, 126 © Foxyliam; p. 31 © aniok; p. 33 © Cat_arch_angel; p. 38 © Hein Nouwens; p. 46 © Kathy Klyopova; p. 48 © umiko; p. 61 © Nata_Alhontess; p. 63 © Sketch Master; p. 67 © B.illustrations; p. 78 © Chailangka; p. 87 © Morphart Creation; p. 95 © Alexander_P; p. 105 © Elena Pimonova; p. 114 © Sabelskaya; p. 116 © Epine; p. 140 © cuttlefish84

NOTE TO READERS: This book has been written and published strictly for informational and educational purposes only. It is not intended to serve as medical advice or to be any form of medical treatment. You should always consult your physician before altering or changing any aspect of your medical treatment and/or undertaking a diet regimen. Do not stop or change any prescription medications without the guidance and advice of your physician. Any use of the information in this book is made on the reader's good judgment after consulting with his or her physician and is the reader's sole responsibility. This book is not intended to diagnose or treat any medical condition and is not a substitute for a physician.

This book is independently authored and published and no sponsorship or endorsement of this book by, and no affiliation with, any trademarked brands or other products mentioned within is claimed or suggested. All trademarks that appear in ingredient lists and elsewhere in this book belong to their respective owners and are used here for informational purposes only. The author and publisher encourage readers to patronize the brands mentioned in this book.

This book is dedicated to my oldest and youngest teachers.

# CONTENTS

**CHAPTER 1: INTRODUCTION** ....................................................1
Caribbean Herbalism Is Storytelling ........................................1
Why Caribbean Herbalism? ......................................................5
Navigating This Book.................................................................8

**CHAPTER 2: ROOTS OF CARIBBEAN HERBALISM** ..................10
Indigenous Roots....................................................................... 11
European Roots ......................................................................... 17
African Roots ............................................................................ 20
Southeast Asian Roots.............................................................. 24

**CHAPTER 3: CARIBBEAN PLANT KNOWLEDGE** .....................27
Aloes (*Aloe vera, A. barbadensis*) ............................................29
Barbadine (*Passiflora quadrangularis*)....................................31
Blue Vervine (*Stachytarpheta jamaicensis, S. cayennensis*) .....33
Bois Canot (*Cecropia peltata*)..................................................35
Cacao (*Theobroma cacao*) ........................................................37
Carpenter Grass (*Justicia pectoralis*) ......................................40
Chadon Beni (*Eryngium foetidum*)..........................................42
Cinnamon (*Cinnamomum* spp.) ...............................................45

Coconut Palm Tree (*Cocos nucifera*)......47

Ginger (*Zingiber officinale*) ......49

Guinea Hen Weed (*Petiveria alliacea*)......51

Lani Bois (*Piper marginatum*)......53

Mango Leaf (*Mangifera indica*)......55

Neem (*Azadirachta indica*)......56

Noni (*Morinda citrifolia*)......58

Nutmeg (*Myristica fragrans*) ......60

Okra (*Abelmoschus esculentus*)......63

Papaya (*Carica papaya*) ......67

Ratchette (*Opuntia cochenillifera*) ......69

Santa Maria (*Lippia alba*)......71

Seriyo (*Sambucus simpsonii*) ......73

Shandilay (*Leonotis nepetifolia*) ......75

Sorrel (*Hibiscus sabdariffa*)......77

Soursop (*Annona muricata*) ......80

Spanish Needle (*Bidens alba, B. pilosa*)......82

Spanish Thyme (*Coleus amboinicus*)......83

St. John's Bush (*Justicia secunda*)......85

Ti-Marie (*Mimosa pudica*) ......87

Turmeric (*Curcuma longa*)......88

Wonder of the World (*Kalanchoe pinnata*) ......91

Zebapique (*Neurolaena lobata*)......92

Some Additional Plants ......95

    Cerasee or Caraili (*Momordica charantia*)......95

    Cotton (*Gossypium* spp.)......95

    Ditay Payee (*Capraria biflora*)......95

    Guava (*Psidium guajava*)......96

    Jigger Bush (*Tournefortia hirsutissima*)......96

    Lime (*Citrus aurantifolia*)......97

    Mat Root (*Aristolochia rugosa*)......97

    Monkey Bone or Firebush (*Hamelia patens*)......97

    Obi Seed or Kola Nut (*Cola nitida*)......97

    Planteh or Plantain (*Plantago major*)......98

    Pussley or Purslane (*Portulaca oleracea*)......98

Roucou (*Bixa orellana*) .......................................................... 98
Seed Under Leaf (*Chanca piedra*) ........................................ 99
Soapvine (*Gouania* spp.) ....................................................... 99
Wild Senna (*Cassia alata*) .................................................... 99

## CHAPTER 4: BUSH TEAS, BUSH BATHS, AND OTHER REMEDIES ................................. 100

Harvesting Medicine .............................................................. 100
Bush Teas ................................................................................ 105
Bush Baths .............................................................................. 108
Root Tonics ............................................................................. 112
Wines ...................................................................................... 113
Tinctures ................................................................................. 114
Oils .......................................................................................... 117

## CHAPTER 5: INTERVIEWS AND BOTANICAL MUSINGS ................. 121

Experiences of a Midwife and Hill Rice Farmer: Alice Prentis ........ 121
Botanical Musings on Genipa .............................................. 126
Dealing with Dengue: From Papaya to Prayers .................. 129
Traditional Wisdom from My Mudda-in-Law: Gloria Parris ........ 134
The Dose Makes the Poison: On Castor Oil and Snake Oil ........ 139

## APPENDIX A: GLOSSARY OF TERMS ................. 144

## APPENDIX B: COMMON AILMENTS AND ASSOCIATED HERBS ...... 146

## APPENDIX C: RESEARCH TIPS ................. 148

## ACKNOWLEDGMENTS ................. 150

## ABOUT THE AUTHOR ................. 152

## CHAPTER 1

# INTRODUCTION

## CARIBBEAN HERBALISM IS STORYTELLING

When I was a child and I was faced with the daunting task of telling someone what I wanted to be when I grew up, I always said that I wanted to be a doctor. Five-year-old me knew that I loved to make people feel better, and I was taught that doctors make you feel better.

From elementary school age, this desire to be a doctor set me up to explore my passion for science and healing. Always a focused and determined child, I signed myself up to join Mensa and to try out for children's *Jeopardy!* I spent summers at STEM (science, technology, engineering, and mathematics) camps, and when I was fourteen, I started working as an aide at the University of Maryland Medical Center. I worked there as an MRI technologist's aide all the way through high school and college, and throughout college I also worked in the neurobehavioral unit at another hospital, Kennedy Krieger Institute. In college, I chose a premed track with a major in physiology and neurobiology.

I say all this to say that I was and am focused on the same goal that has manifested in different ways over the years. My curiosity for understanding God, science, nature, and the human condition has always been insatiable and practical. I research, I practice, I produce repeatable results. I employ the scientific method in my day-to-day life to answer the endless stream of questions and hypotheses running through my mind, whether related to herbs or not. How can we maximize our food-based nutrition throughout the day? What is the mechanism of action of this herb? In which medium are certain nutrients most soluble and bioavailable? How can I mimic nature to make my life more efficient? How can I prove that love has mass and is the true language of God?

As for the last question, I pour my love tangibly into my medicines for my family, and that is also one of the ways through which I hear instructions from the Creator. I am constantly testing this hypothesis and heeding instructions. This manifests in daily life as discovering which plants I can use in my vicinity for various ailments. The goal is to live a healthy lifestyle that does not require much input besides prayer, healthy movement, eating, and hydration. And to create a well-oiled machine that does not need much maintenance. However, life happens, and sometimes you need supplements to support your healing journey.

When this happens, I usually look no further for help than the plants in my yard and neighborhood. I am surrounded by plants that have been used for centuries and studied in modern times for various ailments. The Caribbean and Trinidad are a hotbed of biodiversity and traditional knowledge about useful plants. Because of the widespread Caribbean diaspora, Caribbean herbalism is a broad topic of great interest to people around the world. From ancient history to modern times, plants and herbs have been at the service of humankind. "Herbs for the service of mankind!" is a saying that many Caribbean elders will quote to you, paraphrasing from the Bible:

*"He causeth the grass to grow for the cattle, and herb for the service of man: that he may bring forth food out of the earth."*

Psalm 104:14

Herbs or green plants being at the service of humankind is a key theme of plant–human relationships in the Caribbean. You will find this out quickly during a walk in the bush with a bush man who knows that almost every plant and tree has a use for humans. Some uses are stronger than others, some are more toxic, some are gentler, and some are more effective. But the fact remains that all plants have parts that can be useful.

The beauty of Caribbean herbal knowledge is that it lives in the people. The downside to this is that there is not as much scholarly or published work on the matter. Much as with other Indigenous ways of being, it is mainly an oral tradition passed down from generation to generation. The knowledge lives in your grandmother's heart, your grandfather's hands, and your neighbor's garden. People may not always be able to tell you how or why something works, but they can often give you a list of herbs that either they have used or someone they know has used for an ailment. The knowledge of these plants lives on within everyone. Almost everyone can tell you something about traditional plant medicine, and no one person holds all the knowledge. This is why interviewing people and compiling these stories is an important step in further appreciation of Caribbean folk medicine.

My grandmother, Anastasia May Fraser, turns ninety-six this year, and she is one of my favorite people to talk with about these traditions. Although she has severe dementia, I can still take her into her garden and ask her what a plant is used for. If I am lucky, I will also get information on when to plant it, when to prune it, and when to harvest it. One of the major complaints with our generation and herbal knowledge is that our family members and elders did not pass down everything they knew. This is only partially true.

INTRODUCTION

3

I find that two main issues have caused a break in this transfer of knowledge. The first issue is that we do not spend enough time with elders, asking them questions, building deeper relationships with them, and observing their actions. The moment I start coming around more often and showing love, the floodgates of information open and most people are more than happy to share, once they know that I plan to use the information for the betterment of myself and others. There is often a test involved in this transfer of knowledge, which many people fail. It involves organic reciprocity that an elder may pull out of you without your knowing it. Before you learn about an herb, you may find yourself serving as a chauffeur, a therapist, a laborer in their home or garden, a shoulder to lean on. Until trust is built, you will find that the information given will be superficial at best. Some remedies and healing prayers are shrouded in secrecy, for good reason, and should not be used by just anyone.

The second issue is that even though the current trend is to look for alternative and natural healing modalities, in recent history most of these natural remedies and healing modalities were ostracized and considered less convenient. As a result of development, a lot of the habitats of these plants, along with the plants themselves, are also disappearing. People left behind finicky bush medicines that are hard to find in search of standardized pharmaceuticals that are socially accepted and available at every corner store or pharmacy, all while reminiscing on the days when a good bush bath and bush tea cured every ailment. I find that even when people remember the usefulness of remedies, some feel shy about sharing the virtues of plant medicine because they consider it to be taboo.

A typical conversation with my grandmother about herbs goes like this:

**Me:** "Grandma, what is this plant good for?"

**Grandma:** "Leyaaaa, you know I don't use them things anymore."

**Me:** "Well, what did you used to use it for in the past?"

**Grandma:** "Well, long time people used it for cough and colds. My mother used to boil a few leaves and give to us to clean we out! And we never got sick. Praise God!"

The "praise God" is an important part of her message, which is often forsaken in modern herbal traditions. One consistent thing I have learned from talking with elders is that plants are not divorced from your own spiritual tradition. From Hindu to Orisa to Protestant to Catholic to Islam, calling on the healing power of plants is directly tied to calling on the healing power of God. In a book called *Maljo, Bush Teas and Secret Prayers: Trinidad Cocoa Panyols' Beliefs* by Sylvia Moodie-Kublalsingh, the author details some of the prayers used by powerful healers in Trinidad who mixed Indigenous, African, and Spanish elements in their healing traditions. Prayers are often considered more powerful than herbs, but the herbs can help prayers go to where they need to go.

# WHY CARIBBEAN HERBALISM?

This book is titled *Caribbean Herbalism: Traditional Knowledge and Modern Healing*; however, it can by no means speak for all of the Caribbean. Within the Caribbean there are many cultures, dialects, and languages, and there could be a separate encyclopedia on the herbal traditions of each different Caribbean nation. This book attempts to talk about the common threads within Caribbean herbal traditions and herbs that can be found in a majority of the Caribbean islands and countries.

Geographically, the Caribbean consists of all the islands within the Caribbean Sea and often includes the coastal regions that touch the Caribbean Sea. In terms of diaspora, the Caribbean community reaches around the Earth, with concentrations in places including New York City, Toronto, London, Miami, and Atlanta. Wherever

Caribbean people migrate and congregate, they create rich communities rooted in traditions from their homeland. They open grocery stores that sell the food and fruits from their homeland, they start restaurants that cater to Caribbean taste buds, and they create enclaves to raise their children with shared culture.

Regarding herbal medicine, the Caribbean is a place that should be studied more intentionally. It is well known that many Western medicines come from plants in the Amazon rainforest. It has been found that up to 25 percent of all pharmaceutical drugs come from Amazonian plants. Caribbean islands are right next to and a part of the Amazon River basin, so we have many of the same plants. We also have a unique creolization of herbal medicine practices from Indigenous, African, European, and Southeast Asian influences that takes these medicinal plants and creates unique remedies and traditions borrowed from around the world. A Caribbean tanty, or grandmother, may be calling on traditional Chinese medicine, Ayurveda, European folk

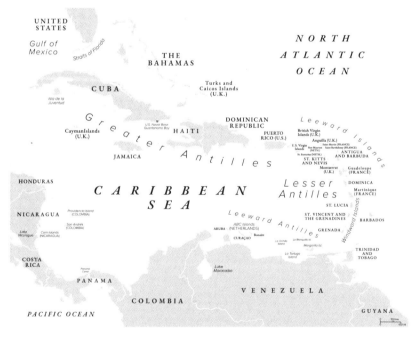

Caribbean Islands

medicine, and African- and Indigenous-based practices while practicing Caribbean herbalism.

I am a product of Trinidadian American culture, and I was raised in Baltimore, Maryland. I come from a family who loved their Trinidadian culture and always hoped that our generation would fully embrace it as well. My childhood memories are interspersed with Carnival hopping in different cities, from Toronto to Miami to Washington, DC. I watched, bright-eyed, from the sidelines as my aunties, uncles, and cousins played Mas (a Trinidadian cultural term which is short for Masquerade and refers to the Carnival procession) in beautiful costumes. In college, I learned to play the steel pan and played in a steel pan orchestra during Carnival celebrations, surrounded by the high energy and sweet tones of my friends on bass and tenor pans and the crowds dancing around us. I can still feel every note on a cellular level as the memories play back in my mind.

We always ate Trinidadian foods and listened to Caribbean music in our household. Holidays were spent with calypso and curry chicken. Packages of Trinidad Cheese and Black Cake were a welcomed gift from visitors. I always understood Carnival and Trinidadian foods as preserving culture. As a diaspora baby, I have always felt it was something I needed to hold on to and claim and nurture. It was my connection from a distance, an umbilical cord of sorts, always pumping calypso and soca through my veins.

Therefore, this book has a Trinidadian perspective, with research and information from other countries, such as Grenada, Guyana, Jamaica, Montserrat, Puerto Rico, Haiti, Saint Lucia, and Barbados. The history of the movement of peoples in the Caribbean speaks to how the same plants and traditions are found in the different nations. From the Indigenous peoples who moved freely between the islands and mainland to the Europeans who colonized the area, every culture is responsible for adding to the tapestry of Caribbean culture with the plants and knowledge that they brought with them.

INTRODUCTION

As you can tell, the Caribbean is a broad topic and a diverse place. A plant that is used in one Caribbean country for every ailment may be considered a roadside weed of little importance in another Caribbean country. The same plant may also be used for different things and in different preparations, depending on the region. In this book, I do not attempt to share every Caribbean healing plant or every use of each plant. This book is grounded in my own experience and research about the region, and it will not shed light on all the nuances of the topic. However, I know that anyone in the Caribbean diaspora will relate to the information in this book, and learn from it as well.

# NAVIGATING THIS BOOK

How to read this book:
- With a curious mind.
- With a pen and paper to take notes.
- With new questions formulating in your mind.
- With the understanding that each concept and plant mentioned could have its own book, and this is just a short distillation of my own research and experiences.
- With the understanding that the author tried her best to speak truthfully, with citations and sources.
- With the understanding that you should research further any herb that you plan to ingest on your own. Do not just take anyone's word for it.
- With the desire to build a personal relationship with the plants in your physical proximity and ancestral lineage.
- With the reminder to be hypervigilant when identifying, foraging, and using herbs. Check and double-check your ID's if you are not sure, because there are poisonous look-alikes out there.

❧ With the reminder that nothing written here is a personal prescription or medical advice.

In this book, I share how and why these herbs work and give anecdotal insights into the culture surrounding their usage. In Chapter 2, I give some background of the cultures, people, and practices that contribute to Caribbean herbalism. In Chapter 3, I give detailed descriptions and uses of select Caribbean herbs that are well known among different islands and countries. These descriptions are interspersed with information from interviews, primary research, and scientific articles about the plants. In Chapter 4, I go over some of the common ways that Caribbean herbs are employed, from bush teas to bush baths to tonics and oils. Finally, in Chapter 5, I share interviews with elders about traditional healing and a few essays of my own.

Please use this book as a reference and a resource but not as a bible! Everything in these pages is there to excite your curiosity and encourage your inner herbalist/scientist/truth seeker to delve deeper than the explanations laid out here. Many of the herbs I discuss can be both healing and toxic. Therefore, they should be treated with reverence and not abused. Traditional medicine has always been a complex dance with life and death, poison and healing potions. The medicine maker and communities held the knowledge of which plant killed and which one healed, and not only which plant but which parts of plants and which dosages created therapeutic effects and not unintended side effects.

This is why I always say that the more you know about plants and people, the less you know! This means moving past the first question of "What's it good for?" or "What can I use for xyz problem?" and really being curious about "How does this plant work?" and "What is the root issue?" It is a lifelong journey to be in right relation with the plants around us, as well as with our own bodies. I believe that nurturing these relationships is key to personal and planetary health!

INTRODUCTION

# CHAPTER 2

# ROOTS OF CARIBBEAN HERBALISM

*"A people without the knowledge of their past history, origin, and culture is like a tree without roots."*

Marcus Garvey

The Caribbean is a deeply creolized culture. The many cultures that have settled on these beautiful shores have spent centuries syncretizing their belief systems and creating new ways of being and knowing. We are most familiar with creolization of language through patois and pidgin, which mix European, African, and Indigenous words and phrases to create island-specific dialects and enabled communication between different groups. In addition to language, there was creolization of herbal medicine practices among the different cultures. Cheryl Lans explained how this played out on the island of Trinidad and Tobago in her book *Creole Remedies of Trinidad and Tobago*.

In this chapter, I share more about the four major cultures that influence Caribbean herbalism. I share how they got to the Caribbean and the plants and plant knowledge that they brought with them. One common theme is that some of this "folk" or "bush" knowledge transcends country of origin, and many practices have shared roots in all four of those major cultures.

# INDIGENOUS ROOTS

The story of Indigenous peoples' movement throughout the Caribbean and the Americas can be traced through plant names and herbal traditions. The first foragers and nomads entered the Caribbean islands from South America over six thousand years ago. Over time, the region would see the influence and settlement of Taino, Kalinago, Warao, Mayan, and other distinct cultures. Much as is true today, the Caribbean has always been a diverse tapestry, woven with different cultures living in both peace and conflict on the seven hundred islands that make up the Caribbean. A large aspect of culture is the plants that people used and carried with them in their nomadic travels.

The earliest inhabitants mainly hunted for their sustenance, utilizing the abundance of wildlife on land and in the sea to sustain their communities. Later, other Indigenous people who settled there utilized a system of agriculture that included crop rotation to ensure the constant supply of staple crops such as cassava (*Manihot esculenta*), sweet potato (*Ipomoea batatas*), arrowroot (*Maranta* spp.), corn (*Zea mays*) and yam (*Dioscorea* spp.). They usually moved plots every two to three years after the soil was depleted, so that they could ensure fertility.[1]

I give special attention to Indigenous roots of Caribbean herbalism because the Caribbean is a deeply colonized and immigrant culture. Often, the contributions of Indigenous cultures are overshadowed by those of African, Southeast Asian, and European cultures. Today, it is hard to always pinpoint where a tradition started, but if you

---

1    Hilary McD. Beckles and Verene A. Shepherd, *Liberties Lost: Caribbean Indigenous Societies and Slave Systems* (Cambridge University Press, 2004).

consider that the majority of plants used in Caribbean herbalism are of neotropical (the Americas) origin, you can see that Indigenous people would have been using them and passing on knowledge of their uses to the newcomers. Many people falsely assume that Amerindians of the Caribbean are extinct, but they are not, and their legacy lives on in the people and the plants of the region.

They also deeply understood the purpose and uses of plants for spiritual, culinary, and medicinal purposes. Lignum vitae (*Guaiacum officinale*) is the national flower of Jamaica, and among the Indigenous Taino population, it was called guayacan, meaning "holy tree." It was a sacred tree used to carve wooden sacraments and to help women's health and sexually transmitted diseases. Some other plants utilized by ancient people that remain important today are cocoa (*Theobroma cacao*); tobacco (*Nicotiana tabacum*); arrowroot (*Maranta arundinacea*); topi tambo (*Calathea allouia*); guanabana (*Annona muricata*), also known as soursop; guava (*Psidium guajava*); genipa (*Genipa americana*); roucou (*Bixa orellana*), also known as annatto; and many others that I detail later in this book.

Indigenous people of the Caribbean also used the trees and plants around them for hunting, shelter, and crafts. For example, a plant in Trinidad called balbac (*Serjania* spp.) is a fish poison; it is placed into water to shock fish, and then the fish are caught as they float downstream. Many different palm species were used for shelter, such as timite (*Manicaria saccifera*), which makes a very strong thatching material. Another plant, in the arrowroot family (Marantaceae), named tirete (*Ischnosiphon arouma*), is used to make fishing baskets and other crafts. These plants are still found throughout the Caribbean, but as a result of deforestation, many of them are slowly disappearing and becoming endangered. Tirete grows only at elevations above two thousand feet, and it prefers humid cloud forests. Ethnobotanists, environmentalists, and Indigenous communities are making efforts to conserve and cultivate these culturally important plants, and I hope books like this will encourage others to do the same.

Although the plants and numbers of Indigenous people have dwindled, the knowledge lives on! Guyana and Suriname are two countries in the Caribbean where there is still a sizable Indigenous population that carries on these traditions. What is interesting about Guyana and Suriname is that they are part of CARICOM (Caribbean Community) intergovernmental organization, but they are on the South American continent instead of within the Caribbean Sea. The populations of these countries are a mix of people of African, Indian, and European descent, but within the interiors, there are still remote villages with people of Warao, Arawak, and Taino ancestry.

Between Trinidad and Tobago, Puerto Rico, Jamaica, and Guyana, I have friends with Indigenous roots who carry on the culture through oral, culinary, and herbal traditions. One beautiful family owns a business called La Flor Traditional Exotics which is based in Guyana and Trinidad. They make and sell traditional goods like cassava bread, farine, cassareep, cocoa tea, chocolate, and carapa (*Carapa guianensis*) seed oil (a.k.a. crab oil or andiroba oil). All the plant products that I just named originated in South America or the Caribbean. Therefore, the safe ways to process them and utilize their medicinal benefits come from centuries of Indigenous peoples' knowledge passed down until today.

Cassava is such an important plant to people all around the world today, even though it originated in South America. It would never have been a staple crop if Indigenous peoples had not found a way to extract the poison from the plant, rendering it safe to eat. Indigenous peoples peeled it, grated it, and then squeezed the liquid out. It was known then that the peels of the cassava and the freshly squeezed liquid should be avoided. Today, it has been shown that bitter cassava contains high concentrations of poisonous cyanide compounds. However, the grated, squeezed, and dried cassava can be used in all manner of dishes, and it can be preserved for long periods of time in the form of shelf-stable farine. Farine is made from grated, crumbled, dried, and then parched cassava bits. It is delicious! The juice can be left to sit for a day, so that the starch settles at the bottom, then poured off and boiled for a long time until it darkens and gains the consistency of molasses. This is cassareep. My great-aunt still has her matapee, a woven cylinder used to squeeze the juice out of cassava through a tugging motion. She uses hers whenever she makes cassava pone!

Indigenous people saw it as important to use and honor a whole plant and as many parts as possible. Nothing should be wasted. Even the poisonous cassava paste was used on spears and arrows for hunting and war. They used pure ingenuity and connection to nature to waste not and want not. Amerindians' relationship with spirits, animals, and plants is not one of dualism. They see humans as kin and allies to the plants and animals in their ecosystem. Plants and animals were to be communed with, and medicine men or shamans were well respected for their ability to contact spirits and know which plants to use for which purposes.

The notion that disease and illness is caused by negative energies and spirits is present in different cultures but especially in Indigenous cultures. This aspect of finding the spiritual root of illness is something you will still see today in the Caribbean. There is a personification of illness within Indigenous and African cultures that implores sick people and healers to seek the human and nonhuman sources of affliction. For example, when my daughter got a fever at eight weeks of age, my grandmother urged me to watch whose energy I allowed in our space and to give the baby a bush bath with sweet broom (*Scoparia dulcis*) to remove any ill intentions.

One thing that I find fascinating is how the vernacular names of plants demonstrate the movement of peoples between regions. Ukee ukee (*Martinella obovata*), a member of the Bignoniaceae family, is a fairly common vine in Trinidad. For generations and generations, it has been one of the most effective cures for conjunctivitis and inflammation of the eyes. Its common name comes from the Arawak family of languages. The plant is native to the Andes and Amazon regions. What is interesting is that although most plants have many uses, this one is almost universally and solely used as a powerful eye medicine. The ethnobotanist Alwyn Gentry found that out of eight countries and thirteen linguistic groups studied, *Martinella obovata* was almost exclusively used as eye medicine, which is rare; most herbs are used or prepared in different ways in different countries and for different ailments. Its use and preparation from Peru to Brazil to Venezuela to Trinidad are noted to be strikingly similar. This means that the ancient knowledge of this plant has been passed down from generation to generation. This fact also speaks to the early contact between South American and Caribbean Indigenous communities.[2]

Its pronunciation is strikingly similar across different countries and regions as well. It has names like yuquilla, lukillia, and yuquillo, depending on the country you are in. These names, as well as the name in the Caribbean, ukee ukee, all have roots in ancient Arawak languages and could possibly show linkages of cultures and the movement of peoples in ancient times. Across Latin America and the Caribbean, users dig up the root, scrape the outer bark, and extract the juice from the pulp of the root. The juice is dripped into the eye and brings almost instant relief.[3]

Although it grows in rainforest margins, it is often planted in the Indigenous home garden for continual and immediate use. I have used ukee ukee to effectively treat conjunctivitis, and whenever my eyes are feeling sore, I will dig some root and make a preparation. It is a slow-growing root that takes years to mature, so you must be careful to dig only a small portion of the root to use at any given time. It is also one of the plants from which I collect seeds and scatter them throughout the forest to repopulate it.

---

2    A. H. Gentry and K. Cook, "*Martinella* (Bignoniaceae): A Widely Used Eye Medicine of South America," *Journal of Ethnopharmacology* 11, no. 3 (1984): 337–43, doi: 10.1016/0378-8741(84)90079-5.

3    Gentry and Cook, "*Martinella* (Bignoniaceae)."

The following is a firsthand account of ukee ukee's Indigenous uses, written in 1791 and published in 1841. I present this as a segue to my discussion of the European influences and roots of Caribbean herbalism.

In traversing the woods of Demerary with my then fellow labourer Mr. Lochhead in 1791, we took up residence in the woods for some days among the wood cutters, the only Europeans or civilized inhabitant that were to be found in those remote parts. One of them was just recovering from a violent inflammation of his eyes. We were solicitous to know what medicines he had found for his relief in a part far remote from medical assistance. He told us his Indian woman was his physician by administering the piece of a common plant in the woods.

We asked him if he would be kind as to show it to us. He told us as he might mistake the plant for others very like it, he would send this Indian woman for some as these men associate and live with Indians in such situations they are at the devotion of the European. In a few minutes the Indian brought the plant to us. We soon learned that it was known to the aborigines time immemorial, and afterwards heard many remarkable accounts of its effects among the Europeans throughout this country, but strange hardly one of them knew the plant being supplied with it by the Indians, nor will these people make known their medicine unless to such people as the wood cutters.[4]

---

4   Gentry and Cook, "*Martinella* (Bignoniaceae)."

CARIBBEAN HERBALISM

# EUROPEAN ROOTS

In the preceding quote, a firsthand account of Europeans learning from Indigenous people about ways to heal their eyes with ukee ukee (*Martinella obovata*), there are several things to be noted. What stands out to me is that there were layers of European society in the so-called New World, and some layers were more trusted than others by Indigenous peoples. The woodcutters and laborers who lived among the First People seemed to be able to learn more about the secrets of plants, and they served as middlemen and liaisons with other Europeans who were there. I have read accounts of Amerindians being tied up and threatened with a poisonous arrow to coerce them to reveal to Europeans the correct plant for the antidote. The plant in this instance is called contrayerva (*Dorstenia contrajerva*).[5]

They guarded this information as sacred, and Europeans pried it out of them using very unsavory methods. This means that the information they got was not always fully correct, but it is the majority of what we have today to understand the history of plant medicines before colonization. It also should be noted that although this information was greatly sought after and is utilized to this day in the making of pharmaceutical drugs, the owners of this knowledge were called uncivilized and savage, all the while healing and feeding the European colonizers.

Cristoforo Colombo landed in present-day Bahamas, Cuba, and Haiti or the Dominican Republic during his first voyage and set off a chain of events that would forever change the world. He was representing Spanish interests, and in the coming centuries, the French, English, Dutch, Scottish, Portuguese, and Irish would all colonize different Caribbean islands at various times. The exchanges that

---

5   Stefanie Gänger, "The Secrets of Indians: Native Knowers in Enlightenment Natural Histories of the Southern Americas," in *Connecting Territories: Exploring People and Nature, 1700–1850*, ed. Simona Boscani Leoni et al. (Brill, 2020), 101–24.

occurred between the Americas, Europe, Africa, and Asia spread people, plants, diseases, violence, knowledge, and religions in ways that would ripple through every society on this Earth.

Even with this checkered history, I lean on these historical accounts from early Europeans in the Caribbean to find out about Indigenous uses and preparations of herbal medicines, dyes, and fibers. Although European cultures destroyed a lot of Indigenous knowledge and practices, they also created some of the only historical written accounts available today. I use the botanical drawings of a Dutch woman, Maria Sibylla Merian, in my research, and I reference the writings and ethnobotanical insights of the region from Sir Hans Sloane. Botanical gardens and herbaria such as the National Herbarium of Trinidad and Tobago are also the legacies of colonial powers. They can be extremely useful, but at the same time they are limited in their scope, and the plant histories have been recorded through a lens of colonial power.

Trinidad and Tobago has one of the most diverse colonial histories in the Caribbean. It was colonized by the Spanish in 1592 and was ceded to Great Britain in 1797. Throughout its history, Trinidad has had Spanish, Dutch, French, and British interests trying to control its people and resources. This is witnessed in creole language, architectural styles, place-names, and local plant names. Many herbs, such as ditay payee (*Capraria biflora*) and bois canot (*Cecropia peltata*), have French creole names. Ditay payee means "tea of the countryside," and bois canot means "canoe wood." The Cocoa Panyol communities of Trinidad still speak Spanish and retain prayers and healing traditions from Spain. Although the official language spoken in Trinidad has changed over the centuries, it is currently English, as a marker of recent British control that was ended in 1962. My last name, Fraser, is an indicator of Scottish Highlander history in my Caribbean bloodline. This is to show that Europe is not a monolith, and each European country had distinct influences on Caribbean culture.

One of the most pervasive aspects of European culture that reached the Caribbean is religion. The majority of Caribbean islanders are

Christian, and more specifically, Roman Catholic. Many cultures around the world more easily adopted Roman Catholicism because its rituals and traditions allowed them to still practice their own animist and nature-based traditions. While in Italy on a pilgrimage visiting sites of Black Madonna worship, I learned that in Europe, many churches were built on top of ancient temples for various goddesses, and Black Madonna festivals lined up with the timing of different pagan festivals.

A large component of Caribbean herbalism is the use of prayers and rituals involving Catholic saints to aid in healing along with plants. Amerindian, African, and Asian cultures syncretized their spiritual practice with Catholic teachings to continue their rituals and not be punished for their beliefs. So, religion played a role in divorcing people from healing traditions, and it also played a role in creating healing traditions that include aspects from different cultures.

In addition to the herbal knowledge from Indigenous people that they documented, Europeans came to the Americas with their own healing traditions, which contributed to the roots of Caribbean herbalism. Their folk system of knowledge included the doctrine of signatures and the humours. The doctrine of signatures is a system of understanding how plants can help humans. It looks at the form of a plant or its "signature" (color, texture, shape) and relates it to its function in the human body. For example, red flowers are considered good for blood, and yellow parts of plants are considered good for jaundice. The four humours, which can be traced to ancient Greece, are blood (heart/air), phlegm (lungs/water), yellow bile (liver/fire), and black bile (spleen/earth). Medieval European doctors would diagnose people on the basis of the perceived imbalance of these four elements. For example, liver issues would be treated with cooling teas and herbs, since liver is related to fire and heat.

Europeans also would have recognized some of the plant families and inferred the uses of plants in different families. Railway daisy (*Bidens pilosa*) is native to the Caribbean, and it is in the Asteraceae family. Asteraceae is a widespread family around the world, with many

ROOTS OF CARIBBEAN HERBALISM

members that are native to Europe, such as dandelion (*Taraxacum officinale*) and the European daisy (*Bellis perennis*). You can see that railway daisy got its name from its resemblance to the European daisy. St. John's bush (*Justicia secunda*) is a New World plant that turns water red. In Europe, St. John's wort (*Hypericum perforatum*) gives a red pigment from its flowers. St. John's bush would have gotten its name from Europeans who noted the similarities.

In addition to these look-alikes, Europeans brought staple food grains such as wheat (*Triticum* spp.) and oats. They also introduced many herbs that are now staples in Caribbean herbalism, including comfrey (*Symphytum officinale*), Irish sea moss (*Chondrus crispus*), parsley (*Petroselinum crispum*), rosemary (*Salvia rosmarinus*), anise (*Pimpinella anisum*), and many others. Some plants grow wild, such as plantain (*Plantago major*). Plantain is not to be confused with the banana relative. It is a broadleaf plant that grows everywhere and is called Englishman's footprint because it can be found throughout the Caribbean and the Americas wherever Europeans walked. According to ethnobotanists Bradley Bennett and Ghillean Prance, in a study of European plants used in South American folk medicine, 38 percent of 216 plants used by respondents had European or Mediterranean origins.[6]

# AFRICAN ROOTS

While noting that Caribbean herbalism started with the first inhabitants of the land, much credit over the years has been given to the strong African influence on the traditional use of plants in the Caribbean and the Americas. Africans came to the Americas with their

---

6   B. C. Bennett and G. T. Prance, "Introduced Plants in the Indigenous Pharmacopoeia of Northern South America," *Economic Botany* 54, no. 1 (2000): 90–102, doi: 10.1007/BF02866603.

own knowledge of plants and growing systems. Judith Carney's *In the Shadow of Slavery* is a great book that outlines the movement of plants and skills throughout the triangular trade. It outlines the botanical legacies of Africans in the Americas by discussing the history of some of the common crops, such as okra (*Abelmoschus esculentus*), watermelon (*Citrullus lanatus*), cowpea (*Vigna unguiculata*), and sorghum (*Sorghum bicolor*). The people indigenous to the Caribbean and the Africans who arrived there had similar ways of relating to the land and plant kin, so their ways of knowing were easily merged to create the basis of Caribbean herbalism.

Both Indigenous and African herbalism focus on bringing harmony and balance into the body and physical environment. They both recognize ancestors and spiritual elements in nature, and they seek to address the mind, body, and spirit as a whole. There is often a medicine man or woman who serves as a conduit between the plants, the person, and the spirit world and who prescribes medicines and performs healing ceremonies, although most people in a community have at least some knowledge of traditional healing. In Cuba there is Santeria; in Haiti there is Voudoun; in Trinidad there are Orisa practitioners. All of these creole religions are based in western African traditions and are still used today. Many people still go to healers based in these systems for divination to gain insight into the reasons for their illness and for treatment options.

Africans in the Caribbean came from the Bight of Biafra, the Gold Coast, the Windward Coast, Sierra Leone, Senegambia, Central Africa, and other areas. This means that they also came with distinct cultures and healing traditions. They often all get lumped in together, but it is important to note that there was creolization of African culture before creolization of Caribbean culture. Although many people believe that the slave trade was purely about labor, it was also about the need for intellectual property and different expertise. Africans came to the Americas as intellectuals, engineers, farmers, and medicine men.

> In colonial times, in the home of the aristocratic white slave owner as in that of the masses of the people, black male and female curanderos [folk healers] rivaled the medical doctor. Their clientele was numerous; their wisdom, or better yet, their natural ability, their "gift," sparked more faith than the awe inspiring science of the university graduate.[7]

There is a famous case of an enslaved man, named Onesimus by his enslaver (who was a prominent minister), who helped bring the science behind vaccinations to the Americas. He was living in Boston during a particularly bad outbreak of smallpox. His enslaver wrote the following in a letter:

> I had from a servant of my own an account of its being practised in Africa. Enquiring of my Negro man, Onesimus, who is a pretty intelligent fellow, whether he had ever had the smallpox, he answered, both yes and no; and then told me that he had undergone an operation, which had given him something of the smallpox and would forever preserve him from it; adding that it was often used among the Guramantese and whoever had the courage to use it was forever free of the fear of contagion. He described the operation to me and showed me in his arm the scar which it had left upon him.[8]

The operation described would have been rubbing pus from a smallpox-infected person into a cut on Onesimus's arm. This was a predecessor to modern vaccines, and although vaccination gives even less exposure to virus, this method did activate immune responses

---

7   Margarite Fernández Olmos, "Black Arts: African Folk Wisdom and Popular Medicine in Cuba," in *Healing Cultures: Art and Religion as Curative Practices in the Caribbean and Its Diaspora*, ed. Margarite Fernández Olmos and Lizabeth Paravisini-Gebert (Palgrave Macmillan, 2001), 29–42.
8   A. Boylston, "The Origins of Inoculation," *Journal of the Royal Society of Medicine* 105, no. 7 (2012): 309–13, doi: 10.1258/jrsm.2012.12k044.

and protected people from disease. It was new to Europeans but well known to Africans at the time.

The African roots of Caribbean herbalism are also witnessed in plant names, practices, and rituals. There is a long list of plant names in the Caribbean starting with the word "Congo." This usually denotes that a plant was either used in or has an analog in African traditional medicine. It may also show that it was historically used by the African population in an area. Some examples are Congo lala (*Eclipta alba*), Congo pump (*Cecropia* spp.), and Congo cane (*Costus* spp.). When Africans came to the Americas, they encountered plants that looked similar to the ones they found at home and had similar actions. Congo lala is a plant that is also found in West Africa, so when Africans came, they saw it and named it Congo lala.

Congo cane is in the *Costus* genus of plants, which is in the ginger family. Different *Costus* species are found native in Africa and the Caribbean, so although they may not have been exactly the same species used in Africa, when people came over they associated them with each other, hence the name Congo cane. According to Dr. Anthony Richards, a Caribbean ethnobotanist, in African Congo culture, the *Costus* species was an insignia of Congo royalty, and it has become an important part of Caribbean medicine and spirituality. In Trinidad, it is used to restore balance to women's wombs, and according to *A Guide to the Medicinal Plants of Coastal Guyana*, it is boiled down with other herbs, like carpenter grass and sorrel, to make cough medicine.[9]

Africans had no choice but to create their own alternative medical systems when they arrived in the Americas and the Caribbean. Many were treated poorly and had very bad living conditions. At the same time, some were free aristocrats and slave owners. Despite the differences in status they were all constantly exposed to disease and violence, which they had to mend themselves because of the same problem as

---

9    Deborah A. Lachman-White et al., *A Guide to the Medicinal Plants of Coastal Guyana* (Commonwealth Secretariat, 1992).

today: expensive, discriminatory health care. Their survival often depended on their ability to use the plant medicine around them and the traditional knowledge from their homelands.

In addition to herbal knowledge, Africans brought their complex spiritual systems that went hand in hand with plant medicine. Both types of knowledge were greatly feared by Europeans, and these African and Indigenous practices were outlawed in many Caribbean countries even after the abolition of slavery and up to the present day. One thing that that colonizers feared was being poisoned. There was a Maroon man from Saint-Domingue named Makandal, who was well known for his esoteric knowledge and political leadership. Although he was executed for his role in rallying Maroons to poison livestock and people to cripple the backbone of the slavery institution, his legacy lived on. People made spiritual herb satchels that they called makandals, which were outlawed shortly after his death in a law that made it illegal for "Negroes to carry makandals or to make and sell drugs."[10]

Today, even though African-based Caribbean spiritual systems such as Voudoun, Obeah, Orisa, Santeria, and Rastafari are still marginalized, there is a beautiful unbroken thread of rituals, prayers, herbs, and oral traditions.

## SOUTHEAST ASIAN ROOTS

The first people from India came to the Caribbean as indentured servants in 1838. They came to present-day Guyana, and in 1845 the first ships arrived with Indians to Trinidad and Jamaica. This movement of people from India to the Caribbean continued until the early 1900s, and as a result, most people of East Indian descent in the Caribbean can trace their ancestry back to the tens of thousands of indentured

---

10    D. Paton, "Witchcraft, Poison, Law, and Atlantic Slavery," *The William and Mary Quarterly* 69, no. 2 (April 2012): 235–64, doi: 10.5309/willmaryquar.69.2.0235.

servants who came during those years. The indentured servitude was meant to last a set number of years, with guaranteed passage back to India. Over time, the length of servitude increased, and Indians were offered pieces of land instead of a return to their homeland. Many took up the offer to stay, and we can thank Indian influence for so much depth of Caribbean culture.

A significant number of Chinese descendants in the Caribbean have also contributed to the culture. Some came as indentured servants, but the majority came between the 1920s and 1940s. Chinese immigrants brought family members over from China as their entrepreneurial endeavors grew. They brought with them a complete system of traditional Chinese medicine. They would have found some familiar herbs in the Caribbean, and they would have brought their own herbs and seeds with them as well.

Indians came to the Caribbean with their own understanding of healing based in Ayurveda and Hinduism. Some of the indentured servants would have been doctors and Brahmans (spiritual healers), who would have introduced those practices to the already creolized Caribbean. My mother-in-law, Gloria Parris, is of East Indian descent and learned many healing traditions from her family and elders. One of those practices is massaging babies and children in a practice called nara. There are also people I have heard referred to affectionately as "man who does rub" or "woman who does rub." The words run together, and they sound like a one-word title of respect for the people in a community who can crack bones and pull veins and nerves back into alignment. They are traditionally Indian, but at this point the traditions have been passed down to all races.

An elder midwife named Miss Alice told me that her seven-day-old baby died of maljo (evil eye). An unwelcome visitor came by who may have been secretly envious of the child. That same day the baby fell ill, and the next day he died in her arms at the doctor's office. From then on, Miss Alice knew maljo was a serious thing and took steps to protect the rest of her children through satchels, oils, and learning how to do

ROOTS OF CARIBBEAN HERBALISM

jharay from Indian elders in her village. Jharay is traditionally done by a priest who says secret prayers over an afflicted person. The person is usually afflicted by a type of maljo. Ingredients like garlic, ginger, turmeric, or cocoyea broomsticks (*Cocos nucifera*) are passed over the person while specific prayers are recited in Hindi. Nowadays, you still hear of people taking their children to pundits and imams when a child is afflicted with serious illness for which modern medicines or bush medicines are not working.

Indians also brought traditional midwifery practices for pregnant and postpartum mothers that are detailed in the book of postnatal women in Trinidad by Kumar Mahabir. My mother-in-law was of great help during my postpartum period. She reminded me to keep my feet warm, to stay in bed and rest for as long as possible, to drink plenty of turmeric tea, and to eat nourishing meals. She came to our home and helped us with cooking, cleaning, and taking care of the baby so that I could properly heal. Proper postpartum care is a huge part of Caribbean tradition, but it is being lost with new generations.

Southeast Asians have also left a very strong botanical legacy in the Caribbean; a large percentage of our herbal remedies and wild plants can be traced back to Southeast Asia. Popular plants including mango, turmeric, ginger, black pepper, tulsi (*Ocimum sanctum*), dungs fruit (*Ziziphus mauritiana*), banana, and many others. Indian immigrants would have brought these plants to plant in their gardens, and they would have also been a part of the triangular trade between Asia, Africa, and the Americas. Botanical museums and herbaria also would have spread Southeast Asian seeds to the Caribbean. Many of the trees that dot the Queen's Park Savannah in the capital city of Trinidad have roots in Asia and were planted around the savannah for research purposes. The similarities in climates meant that scientists and farmers often wanted to test Indian plants on Caribbean soil.

## CHAPTER 3

# CARIBBEAN PLANT KNOWLEDGE

In these times of fast information, social media, and artificial intelligence, it is very important for people to be able to learn about plants from trusted places. It is imperative to be able to recognize plants and correctly identify them to obtain accurate information about them. In describing each plant, I give botanical characteristics that can be used along with pictures to help you identify an herb. I provide correct Latin names to help you with research and a list of common names from different places.

It is very easy to succumb to confirmation bias when learning about herbs. You might see a social media graphic that promises to treat an issue you are dealing with, or you might be on a hike and see a plant look-alike, assuming it is the same plant you are interested in. Therefore, it is important to take your time with herbal studies and plant identification. Misidentifying herbs or using the wrong herbs for your body or your condition can have negative consequences.

It can be dangerous to self-diagnose a condition and treat it with herbs without solid research or a trusted practitioner guiding your herbal regimen. Be wary of grand claims of cures or miraculous healing from any herb. Many herbs can be just like Western pharmaceuticals in that they can induce negative side effects and should be taken with caution. See my essay "The Dose Makes the Poison" in Chapter 5 for more information about the fine line between medicine and poison.

My hope is that you will read about these plants and be curious enough to do more research, ask more questions, and build your own relationships with them. Do not take the words in this book as fact. They are a collection of experiences, research, and documentation of firsthand knowledge from my community. These anecdotal experiences give you an idea of the power and medicinal action of these herbs, but they are not a personal prescription for you.

I start each plant monograph with the Latin name and common names. The lists of common names are not an extensive list. The same plant can have many different common names within the same country and across a region. Also, one common name could be used for several different plants. These distinctions are especially important in the Caribbean, as we talk to each other about plants, so that we can be sure we are speaking about the correct species.

Under the headings "Traditional Knowledge and Modern Research," you will find information from trusted resources and people about the preparation and plant parts used, as well as the ailments they are used for. Exact quantities are rarely specified, but general guidelines are given throughout. I also share how modern phytochemical research has caught up with traditional knowledge by describing the constituents that have been found, isolated, and tested in these plants.

Visit www.caribbeanherbalism.com to see photographs of the plants mentioned in this book.

# ALOES
*Aloe vera, A. barbadensis*

## Botanical Description

*Aloe vera* or *Aloe barbadensis* is a succulent plant that has thick leaves filled with a translucent gel. The leaves grow around the stem in a rosette pattern. They are green or gray-green, sometimes have white spots, and often have spikes along the outer edges. One interesting thing about the root system is that a type of fungus lives symbiotically on the roots to help the plant extract more nutrients from the soil.

## Traditional Knowledge and Modern Research

Aloes are a staple in many Caribbean gardens and households. Aloe is an ancient plant used for thousands of years throughout Asia, Africa, Europe, and the Americas. In Indian Ayurveda, it is known to keep the body youthful, and in traditional Chinese medicine it is known as bitter and cooling. In the Caribbean, it is used extensively as a remedy for bug bites, burns, and skin abrasions. It is also a well-known purgative and blood cleanser. In Trinidad, a remedy from herbalist Albertina Pavy states to take charcoal powder, aloes, and molasses at the end of an illness to cleanse and purge the system. This was also her remedy for worms and parasites.[11] In order to remove some of the bitter compounds, to which some people are allergic, it is recommended to soak or drain aloes with the cut stem in a cup for an hour before using.

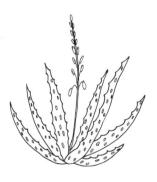

Aloe vera

---

11   Albertina Pavy, *Treatments & Cures with Local Herbs* (Paria, 1987).

Aloe is a common ingredient in many over-the-counter medicines and products. It is one of the most commercialized and industrialized medicinal plants in the world. Over seventy-five medicinally active compounds have been found in aloe, and research now focuses on how to preserve the medicinal actions of these compounds through different processing methods.[12]

## Personal Accounts

*Aloe vera* is the perfect plant for everyone to grow in their home or garden because it does well indoors. It is the ultimate first aid remedy because the gel can be placed on bites or burns and then the green skin can be used as a bandage. I rub the gel from inside the leaves directly on my face to help refresh my skin. I also scoop the gel out and blend it with water, oils, and ratchette (*Opuntia* spp.) as a hair conditioner. I remember the power I felt to heal myself as a young child when I was tasked with breaking off a piece of *Aloe vera* and putting it on my bug bites. Something that stands out about it is that I grew up seeing it at my grandmother's house in Omaha, Nebraska, as well as my grandmother's house in Trinidad and Tobago. This speaks to how important it is to different cultures. I am pretty clumsy and get burns on the stove often enough. I have found that aloe and activated charcoal mixed into a paste provides instant relief from pain and helps my burns not to blister. I am continually shocked at how a minor burn can be healed within a day with this mixture.

---

12   W. J. Martínez-Burgos et al., "*Aloe vera*: From Ancient Knowledge to the Patent and Innovation Landscape—A Review," *South African Journal of Botany* 147 (July 2022): 993–1006, doi: 10.1016/j.sajb.2022.02.034.

# BARBADINE
*Passiflora quadrangularis*
Common names: giant granadilla, badea, grenadine

## Botanical Description

Barbadine is a vine in the passionflower and passion fruit family that is indigenous to the Caribbean and tropical Americas. Its fruit is large, green, and oblong, with thick flesh and hundreds of seeds in the middle that are encased in a slightly sweet-and-sour pulp. As the fruit ripens, it turns yellow and the flesh gets softer. The taste is similar to, but much milder than, that of the more popular passion fruit *Passiflora edulis*, to which it is closely related. The fruit of *Passiflora edulis* is smaller and rounder, with less flesh and more pulp.

## Traditional Knowledge and Modern Research

Barbadine is used for its fruits, flowers, and leaves. The unripe green fruit can be eaten as a vegetable, and when it is soft and yellow, it is traditionally used in a drink called barbadine punch. The leaves and flowers are also made into a medicinal tea used for expelling parasites and as a mild sedative. It is advised not to drink too much of it or drink it too often because it has effects similar to a narcotic. In Guyana, it is widely used as an antiparasitic treatment for pets. Mr. Balkarran, a host and tour guide in Guyana, told me he puts a strong tea of it in his dogs' drinking water for three days once a year. He said that after three days, "you should see what does come out!"

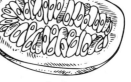
Barbadine

I did not create a separate section about passion fruit, but it has similar uses in that its flowers and leaves are a popular addition to teas to aid in sleep and calming the nerves. Passionflower, soursop, and blue vervine can be combined in a tea for a maximum calming effect on the nervous system to help a person sleep. Passionflower can have a strong effect on the system if taken in high doses, so it is best to start with smaller amounts and work your way up.

## Barbadine Punch

The seed pulp has a lot of flavor, so in order to release some of that flavor into the punch, be sure to save the seeds and follow the instructions in Step 3.

- 1 soft, ripe yellow barbadine fruit
- 3 cups coconut milk
- 5 tablespoons sweetener of choice
- ½ teaspoon nutmeg
- ½ teaspoon cinnamon
- 1 teaspoon tonka bean or vanilla
- 2 dashses Angostura bitters

**Step 1:** Cut the fruit in half, scoop out the seeds in the middle, and set the seeds aside.

**Step 2:** Peel the skin from the outside of the fruit and put the peeled fruit in a bowl.

**Step 3:** Soak the seeds in enough water to cover for 2 to 3 minutes. Then massage the seeds with your fingers and strain the water into the bowl containing the peeled fruit.

**Step 4:** Blend the fruit and the pulp water along with the coconut milk, sweetener, spices, and Angostura bitters. Taste and adjust the levels of sweetener, spices, and bitters to your liking.

**Step 5:** Enjoy over ice or blend with ice for a frozen treat.

# BLUE VERVINE

*Stachytarpheta jamaicensis, S. cayennensis*
Common names: blue porterweed,
rattail vervine, wild vervain

## Botanical Description

Blue vervine is an annual and sometimes perennial member of the Verbenaceae family that is indigenous to South America and the Caribbean. It has attractive serrated oval leaves and long flower stalks that pop out pink, purple, or blue flowers. It is a favorite of hummingbirds and pollinators. Two slightly different species, *Stachytarpheta jamaicensis* and *Stachytarpheta cayennensis*, are used interchangeably and have the same common names in the countries where they are grown. Although blue vervine is also called wild vervain or wild verbena because of similarities in appearance, it is completely different from North American vervains, which are in the *Verbena* genus. This is an example of Latin names being helpful in differentiating between plants with the same or similar common names. As an herbal practitioner or researcher, it is important to be certain of the plant in question and to interrogate whether the common name, the specimen, and the Latin name all belong to the same plant before using it.

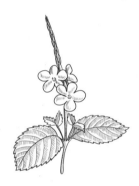

Blue vervine

## Traditional Knowledge and Modern Research

One of the most common traditional uses of this plant in the Caribbean is for postpartum mothers, to increase their milk supply and restore balance to their womb. It also has a strong tradition of use in a tea for gastrointestinal issues, coughs, and colds. The leaf juice or tea is also used in cases of intestinal parasites, where it might be paired with worm grass (*Chenopodium ambrosioides*) and taken for a few days. It is a versatile herb and considered generally safe, so it is a common addition to daily bush tea. However, because of its effects on the uterus, it is not recommended for pregnant women, as it can cause abortion. Finally, an elder Jamaican man once repeatedly told me, "Vervine is a nervine," to emphasize that it calms the nervous system.

All of the traditional knowledge about this plant has been corroborated by modern research. Most of the traditional uses have been attributed to the relatively high presence of healing compounds including alkaloids, tannins, and saponins present in all parts of the plant.[13]

## Personal Accounts

I have blue vervine growing all around my house as an always welcomed "weed" that is there whenever I need it. I put it in nighttime bush teas to help myself settle in for the night. I usually pick five to ten small leaves per cup, along with other herbs like soursop. When I was breastfeeding, although I never had a problem with supply, I drank this weekly because many different women advised me that it would help with postpartum healing and milk production. It is my favorite plant to gift to pregnant women so they can plant it in the ground while they are pregnant and then harvest and use it when breastfeeding. I love eating it raw as I take walks because it has a slightly bitter, slightly sweet taste. The tiny flowers have a slight umami flavor and a taste that is reminiscent of mushrooms.

---

13   P. M. Liew and Y. K. Yong, "*Stachytarpheta jamaicensis* (L.) Vahl: From Traditional Usage to Pharmacological Evidence," *Evidence-Based Complementary and Alternative Medicine* (January 26, 2016): 7842340, doi: 10.1155/2016/7842340.

# BOIS CANOT
*Cecropia peltata*
Common names: Congo pump, trumpet tree

## Botanical Description

Bois canot is a very common tree in the Caribbean that is also native to the region. Its most striking feature is its large leaves, which can vary greatly in size. They are slightly silver or grayish, and their undersides have brownish-reddish ridges. The fruit is edible for humans and is highly attractive to bats and birds. Bois canot is an important part of the ecosystem, and as a pioneer species it is one of the first trees to appear in a disturbed habitat, growing rapidly and providing the ground cover necessary for the survival of less hardy plant species. It is an ideal species to use in the beginning of a land reclamation or reforestation program. The trees are short-lived, rarely lasting more than twenty years, but they greatly benefit the local ecology in their life cycle. They almost continuously produce flowers and fruits that are staple foods for many bird and mammal species.

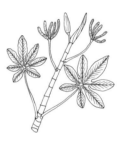

Bois canot

## Traditional Knowledge and Modern Research

The name bois canot is a product of Trinidad and Tobago's French legacy, and it translates literally to "canoe wood." It is pronounced *bwa-ca-no* or *bah-ca-no*. When I was in Guyana, I learned that it is also called Congo pump and it is one of the more common traditional remedies for back pain and kidney issues. There are two closely related species of *Cecropia*. The reddish-stemmed ones are regarded as female and the white-stemmed ones as male, in Guyana. In Trinidad, the green leaves are used as a shampoo and the dried leaves are collected from the ground under trees to be used in teas. The tea is drunk to help with hypertension and diabetes. The tea is also high in mucilage, so it is commonly used for soothing the respiratory tract when someone has a cough or asthma.

## Personal Accounts

Bois canot was probably one of the first trees I could identify with confidence. I remember that one always grew across the street from my grandmother's house in South Oropouche, Trinidad. My childhood Maryland-based brain thought it looked like it was from a Dr. Seuss book! There was a man named Sarge who would harvest the leaves and wash his hair under the standpipe with them. This memory always stuck with me, and it really piqued my curiosity about the power and the uses of the plants around me.

Fast-forward to today, when I am surrounded by bois canot. Matter of fact, everyone in Trinidad has almost a 100 percent chance of passing a bois canot tree at least weekly. In our home, we drink bois canot tea regularly as an ingredient in our bush teas. I once drank too much of it, and I can attest to its effects on blood pressure. I have a blood pressure machine at home and felt my body responding to drinking a strong tea of bois canot, so I took my pressure and noticed it was very low! It was not dangerously low, but it was very noticeable. So, if you are taking blood pressure medication or have chronically low blood pressure, take with caution. Whenever there is Sahara dust in the air, we drink bois canot tea to soothe our throats and lungs.

# CACAO
*Theobroma cacao*
Common names: cocoa, kawkaw

## Botanical Description

Cacao, or the tree that produces cocoa and chocolate, is native to the Amazon and Orinoco River basins. It is a small tree with large oval-shaped leaves with noticeable veins. The flowers are small and delicate, with the five sepals indicative of its place in the mallow or Malvaceae family. From these small flowers, which are pollinated by small midges, large football-shaped fruits are produced. The fruits can range in color from yellow to burgundy to orange when fully ripe, and they have thick skins. Inside the fruit (cocoa pod) are forty to sixty cocoa beans encased in sweet white pulp. The flowers and pods grow directly off the tree trunk and branches. There are three main varieties of cacao, named criollo, trinitario, and forastero. Trinitario is a cross of criollo and forastero, and it originated on the island of Trinidad and Tobago.

## Traditional Knowledge and Modern Research

In cacao's Latin name, *Theobroma* comes from the Greek words "theos," meaning "God," and "broma," or "food." This name was given by Carl Linnaeus in 1753. While *Theobroma* translates as food of the gods, cacao is based on the Olmec word kakaw, retained by the Spanish colonizers of Mesoamerica to describe the tree and what it produces. Since ancient times, cacao has been revered for its sacredness and healing ability. It was a staple in Mayan households, most likely because it is very nutritious and provides many vitamins and minerals and calories needed to maintain health. It was traditionally mixed with honey, corn, and spices such as cayenne pepper to make a frothy drink. The Aztecs called this drink xocoatl, "bitter water," which speaks to

CARIBBEAN PLANT KNOWLEDGE

the bitterness of the beans and tea. In some cultures, cacao is used to treat asthma because of the vasodilating effects of the theobromine molecule (which acts like caffeine but without causing a crash).

In the Caribbean, cacao is usually enjoyed as cocoa tea. Most cocoa beans were historically shipped to northern and European countries to be processed into chocolate, and the lower-grade beans were left behind in the countries of origin. Those beans were ground and mixed with spices like cinnamon, tonka bean, nutmeg, bay leaf, and clove to make a block of coarse chocolate that could be grated into water or milk to make a delicious and nutritious drink. This contrasts with hot chocolate, which is made with cocoa powder instead of the whole cocoa bean. This traditional cocoa tea helped sustain many hungry bellies and greatly reduced malnutrition in Caribbean households by supplementing sparse diets during hard economic times.

Chocolate and cacao beans were always known to be healthy, but in the past decade there has been a renewed appreciation in the media for the benefits of dark chocolate. This has resulted in small-scale artisanal chocolate makers differentiating themselves from large producers like Hershey's and Cadbury by being fair to farmers and carefully selecting beans for quality.

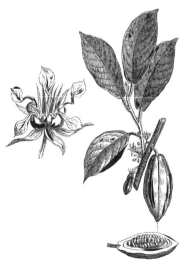

Cacao plant and flower

Cacao is a vasodilator, meaning it widens your blood vessels, especially those in your heart, lungs, and brain. This increases blood flow to those organs and sends whatever other medicine you are ingesting to those areas. Cacao lowers blood pressure and regulates heart rhythm. It is truly a heart-opening experience! It also has strong effects on mood as a result of its theobromine and compounds that mimic cannabinoids, which bind to the cannabidiol receptors in the brain for overall mood enhancement. It is rich in nutrients including iron and magnesium, which also contribute to a sense of well-being and satiation.

## Personal Accounts

*Theobroma cacao* is an intimate part of my life because my husband, Michael Parris, is a chocolatier. We also own an estate that used to be a cacao farm, which we are rehabbing to provide our business, Panorama Cacao, with cocoa beans. We purchase from farmers in the Maracas Valley in Trinidad, where we live, as well as from farmers in Rio Claro, Trinidad. I can fully attest to the heart-opening and warming effects of chocolate; I often joke that was how my husband hooked me! My favorite product of his, Mayan Style Brewing Cacao, is made with fermented unroasted beans that are ground to the consistency of coarse coffee and brewed like coffee. I like to add cinnamon and cayenne pepper and a little honey, and the energy and nutrients it provides can sustain me for a whole day. It is one of my favorite drinks when I am fasting. Most people who eat our 92 percent or 100 percent dark chocolate or who taste the Mayan Style Brewing Cacao speak of how it elevates their mood and makes them feel "warm and fuzzy." My daughter does not eat chocolate, which is good for us; otherwise, we might go out of business! However, she loves eating the sweet pulp of the cocoa beans. I let her do this, especially when she has a cough, to soothe her throat with the mucilage from the pulp, which has bronchodilating effects.

CARIBBEAN PLANT KNOWLEDGE

# CARPENTER GRASS
*Justicia pectoralis*
Common names: carpenter bush, toyeau, tilo, chamba, curia

## Botanical Description

This herb is in the Acanthaceae family and grows low on the ground in shaded, wet areas like forest creeks and drains. It sets new roots as it grows and can easily be harvested and transplanted using pieces with roots on them. The glossy, dark green leaves are pointed and perfectly opposite, forming a cross when viewed from above. The flowers are very small, can be white or purplish white, and look like orchids. Seen along forest creeks and often planted in house yards, carpenter grass is highly aromatic; its crushed leaves release a vanilla-like smell because of the presence of coumarin.

## Traditional Knowledge and Modern Research

This plant received the genus name *Pectoralis*, a Latin word pertaining to the chest, because of its strong action on chest colds and the lungs. Indigenous cultures from Peru to Brazil to Venezuela to the Caribbean have had a special relationship with carpenter grass and planted it in home gardens for ease of access. A handful of these plants can be boiled in water to release their healing properties. The tea is used for coughs and colds and as a mild sedative to reduce anxiety. Another traditional method of preparation is to boil it down with sugar and water to make a cold-medicine syrup that is a good expectorant. Some herbs people in Guyana pair it with are lemongrass (*Cymbopogon citratus*), Santa Maria (*Lippia alba*), daisy (*Wedelia trilobata*), or sweet sage (*Lantana camara*). Carpenter bush also has some psychoactive properties; some ancient Indigenous cultures of South America juiced it to drop in the eyes or powdered it to use as a snuff.[14]

The traditional uses of *Justicia pectoralis* have been corroborated by modern research. Analysis of its constituents shows that it is high in coumarin, which for the plant acts as a defense mechanism against pathogens but for humans acts a biologically active healing compound. Coumarin is found in modern vanilla substitutes, and it is a highly effective anticoagulant (blood thinner), so it should be used with caution. A 2017 scientific article stated that *Justicia pectoralis* "has several biological effects, including its therapeutic potential for the treatment of inflammatory diseases, such as asthma. However, the development of new researches on *J. pectoralis* through modern pharmaceutical technologies and analytical protocols is essential to assure its quality. In addition, a strong collaboration between preclinical and clinical studies is still necessary for the development of an herbal medicine from aerial parts of *J. pectoralis*. These additional researches on *J. pectoralis* will offer a noticeable socio-economic impact enabling the development of a new medicine from this species."[15]

## Personal Accounts

This is one of my mother-in-law's favorite herbs. It reminds her of her childhood, when her mother used it for many ailments and as a general wellness tea. A patch of carpenter grass near her childhood home has been growing there for decades. She likens it to chamomile in its cure-all effects and its calming nature. I also heard about it from

---

14   M. Kujawska et al., "The Relation Between Ashaninka Amazonian Society and Cultivated Acanthaceae Plants," *Economic Botany* 77, no. 4 (2023): 372–409, doi: 10.1007/s12231-023-09585-8.

15   L. K. A. M. Leal et al., "*Justicia pectoralis*, a Coumarin Medicinal Plant Have Potential for the Development of Antiasthmatic Drugs?," *Brazilian Journal of Pharmacology* 27, no. 6 (November–December 2017): 794–802, doi: 10.1016/j.bjp.2017.09.005.

a friend, named Basant, whose favorite tea is a mix of carpenter grass, lemongrass, and cocoa mint (*Peperomia rotofundila*). You can use a handful of carpenter grass, one or two sprigs of lemongrass, and a small handful of cocoa mint. Lemongrass can easily overpower the flavor of a tea, so it's important not to use too much if you want the flavor of the other herbs to come through. I have noticed that to effectively release its active compounds, I can boil the carpenter bush for a few minutes and then place other herbs in the pot with it to steep. The taste of coumarin and vanilla warms you from within and gives an almost instant sense of well-being.

# CHADON BENI
*Eryngium foetidum*
Common names: culantro, fit weed, bandhaniya, recao, spirit weed

## Botanical Description

Chadon (pronounced *shadow*) beni is a striking plant with stiff, shiny, light to dark green spined leaves that grow in a rosette around the stem. They can be almost twelve inches long. The leaves are serrated, and so is the very spiky seed head. It is in the same family (Apiaceae) as coriander and cilantro, and the whole plant has a similarly pungent odor, as noted by *foetidum* in the Latin name.

## Traditional Knowledge and Modern Research

Chadon beni is a popular seasoning and herbal medicine throughout Central and South America and the Caribbean. One of its most common names in Trinidad is bandhaniya, a word borrowed from Hindi. It is one of the main ingredients of green seasoning, which is a delectable and nutritious blend of fresh spices including chadon beni, pimento peppers, garlic, ginger, and chives. This is the base of most dishes, and different Caribbean islands have different versions of the same versatile seasoning. Plants with pungent odors are often seen as helpful in expelling harmful spirits. Epilepsy was once thought to be of a spiritual nature, and this plant was used in Jamaica to calm seizures. This is why it is also known as spirit weed and fit weed. One way to administer this is to soak the leaves and roots in coconut oil and then rub the liquid on the body, especially the temples. It is also traditionally drunk as a tea containing only leaves or leaves and roots.

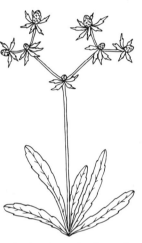

Chadon beni (culantro)

Studies involving animals have clearly demonstrated that chadon beni leaf extracts can expel parasites, reduce convulsions during seizures, reduce inflammation, and function as an anti-inflammatory. The main essential oil of the plant is eryngial, which is being studied extensively in the pharmaceutical industry. There is already a patent for its use in deworming drugs for mammals, including humans.[16]

## Personal Accounts

It was always fun for me to pick the chadon beni from my grandmother's yard in Trinidad for meal prep. I would pick a few leaves if she just wanted to add it to the saltfish or smoked herring for breakfast. I would pick handfuls if she wanted to make green seasoning or pepper sauce. I grew up in Maryland, where we did not have much access to

---

16   J. H. A. Paul et al., "*Eryngium foetidum* L.: A Review," *Fitoterapia* 82, no. 3 (April 2011): 302–8, doi: 10.1016/j.fitote.2010.11.010.

quality chadon beni, so we substituted cilantro from the grocery store, but it never gave the depth of flavor of Trinidad chutneys, peppers, and sauces attributable to chadon beni. I once visited an elder traditional midwife, Alice Prentis, while I was pregnant, and she warned me about using too much of this herb in the weeks leading up to labor but said I should drink the tea of the roots regularly during the week after birth to help with any hemorrhaging.

## Green Seasoning

Each family's green seasoning will have its own unique taste and will be based on what is available. Some people make it shelf-stable by adding salt; some add vinegar or oil. The main ingredients are always chadon beni, garlic, chives, Spanish thyme, and pimento peppers. Here is my family's recipe. It is used as a marinade for meat and as an addition to most curries, stews, and soups. The recipe does not include oil or vinegar, so it is best stored in the refrigerator or in freezer cubes.

about 2 cups chadon beni, rough chopped
1 stalk celery, chopped
about 20 cloves garlic, peeled
1 bunch green onions or chives, sliced
10 leaves Spanish thyme leaves only
5–10 pimento peppers, chopped
1 small knob ginger, sliced
2–3 teaspoons sea salt, or to taste
½ cup water
¼ cup vinegar or lime juice

Place all of the ingredients in a blender and blend to a fine, minced consistency. Bottle and refrigerate.

# CINNAMON

### *Cinnamomum* spp.

*"Take thou also unto thee principal spices, of pure
myrrh five hundred shekels, and of sweet cinnamon
half so much, even two hundred and fifty shekels, and
of sweet calamus two hundred and fifty shekels."*

Exodus 30:23, King James Version

## Botanical Description

The cinnamon tree is a small tree native to Sri Lanka but is grown in tropical regions around the world. There are a few different species. There is the *Cinnamomum cassia* tree, which produces a darker brown and harder bark. The *Cinnamomum verum* (also known as Ceylon cinnamon) tree has a lighter brown and softer bark. The latter is more common in Caribbean islands such as Grenada, where it is a major export. The Ceylon species has a lighter flavor and is not as spicy as the *cassia* variety. Cinnamon is in the laurel family with Mediterranean bay leaf (*Laurus nobilis*), and so its leaves are also used in food and medicine.

## Traditional Knowledge and Modern Research

The quoted Bible verse speaks to the fact that cinnamon has been used as a spice and healing herb for millennia. The passage details the ingredients for an anointing oil that Yahweh provided to Moses. This points to the spiritual healing use of cinnamon in ancient history. It is one of the spices that drove the Arab spice trade that connected Asia and Europe and eventually led to the search for spices in other parts of the world. Cinnamon is a spice that would have been known to African,

East Indian, and European people who settled in the Caribbean. It was introduced to the New World and to the Amerindian people and has been deeply embraced.

Cinnamon is traditionally used as a food additive for flavoring and as a tea and fragrance oil. It has warming effects and helps with blood circulation. It is a comforting spice with an aroma that cultures around the world have embraced in holiday and comfort foods and drinks such as sorrel, cakes, and punches. It is often an ingredient in muscle and joint salves and natural toothpastes because it has pain-relieving and antiseptic properties.

In modern times, cinnamon can be found in essential oils and powdered supplements. It is very popular in health supplements that are added to recipes for cinnamon's antioxidant effects and positive effects on cardiovascular health.

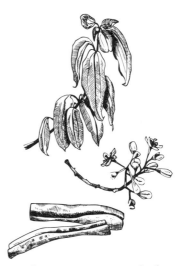

*Cinnamomum verum* leaf, flower, and dried bark

## Personal Accounts

Cinnamon is a must-have ingredient in our household. We buy it from the herb sellers at markets, with their clear plastic bags containing measured portions of barks, seeds, roots, leaves, and powders. I personally like what Trinidadians call "spice," which comes from Grenada and is more often the Ceylon cinnamon variety than the *cassia* variety. We put it in our spice grinder as needed and add it to oatmeal, cocoa tea, smoothies, coffee, soups, baked goods, body salves, chocolate bars, you name it. For healing, I like to make a broth tea with homemade beef bone broth, cinnamon, ginger, turmeric, and nutmeg when I feel a cold or stomach illness coming on.

# COCONUT PALM TREE
*Cocos nucifera*
Common names: water nut, copra

## Botanical Description

The coconut is part of the Arecaceae family, also known as the palm tree family. There are many members of this family with edible and medicinal uses, but coconut is the most popular worldwide. Even though it has "nut" in its name, it is actually a drupe, or a stone fruit. The coconut originated in the Pacific and Indian Ocean basins but spread around the world through trade and colonialism. It grows up to 100 feet tall and can yield dozens of fruits per year. The name comes from the Portuguese "coco" ("skull") because the three dots on a dehusked coconut shell resemble two eyes and a mouth.[17] Coconuts enjoy well-drained soil such as sand, which is why you will often find them on beaches.

## Traditional Knowledge and Modern Research

Most of the traditional knowledge about coconuts comes from the Caribbean's Southeast Asian populations because the coconut was brought to the Americas from that part of the world. In those regions, it has names like tree of life, tree of abundance, or three generations tree to signify its importance to the people who depend on it for survival.[18] Coconut water is used for drinking; dried coconut "meat" is used for food and oil; the branches make brooms, fibers, and baskets; the shell makes household utensils; and the roots are used in herbal

17    Harper Douglas, "Etymology of coco," *Online Etymology Dictionary*, accessed February 7, 2025, https://www.etymonline.com/word/coco.
18    U. Ahuja, "Coconut—History, Uses, and Folklore," *Asian Agri-History* 18, no. 3 (2014): 221–48.

CARIBBEAN PLANT KNOWLEDGE

medicine. Coconut water is known to be hydrating and high in vitamins and minerals. It is drunk during illness, especially gastrointestinal illness, to replenish the body. The oil is known to be antimicrobial and is used to treat skin problems, particularly fungal issues. The root can be made into tea to treat diarrhea and support healing of skin diseases such as rashes and eczema.

Modern studies have tried to verify all of the amazing health claims of coconut oil and water. It has been found to increase metabolism, lower cholesterol, and decrease symptoms of menopause in women. Coconut sugar is considered to have a low glycemic index and can be used by people suffering from diabetes. Coconut oil in its unrefined and virgin state is highly beneficial because of the presence of lauric acid, which studies have shown to be antibacterial and antiviral. Lauric acid in coconut oil is similar to the fats in mother's milk.[19]

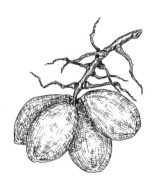

Coconuts

## Personal Accounts

I am blessed to live surrounded by coconuts on my homestead. And when we do not have coconuts, a neighbor will always have one. It is a love language among our neighbors to leave coconuts for others when any of us has an abundance. While pregnant with my daughter, I was encouraged to drink coconut water often to make the baby healthy and have clear skin. Another staple in my house besides coconut water is coconut milk. We make fresh coconut milk at least once a week and use it to cook curry corn and dumplings or callaloo. We also use it in our signature vegan hot chocolate made with our homemade chocolate, spices from the land, and freshly made coconut milk. My husband

---

19   Ahuja, "Coconut—History, Uses, and Folklore."

taught me how to make coconut oil for the first time, and I like to use homemade coconut oil more than the store-bought oil when I am making herbal infusions.

# GINGER

*Zingiber officinale*
Common name: ginger

## Botanical Description

The most-used part of ginger is the golden-tan rhizome that grows underground. The plant has a stem with spear-shaped leaves. It is found in wet, rainy regions. It is easily grown by planting pieces of the rhizome, which will multiply and grow. The leaves and rhizomes are both fragrant.

## Traditional Knowledge and Modern Research

Ginger is a favorite herb in many Caribbean households and around the world. It originated in Asia and would have been popularized in the Caribbean by Indian and Asian migrants and traders. In traditional Chinese medicine, ginger is used for its respiratory (expectorant), gastrointestinal (antinausea), and circulatory (stimulant) effects. It is a warming herb that stimulates blood flow and perspiration. In Indian Ayurvedic medicine, ginger is seen as a digestive tonic that is useful for difficult digestion. These uses have been passed down through the ages throughout different cultures. Here in the Caribbean, it is regularly used in the treatment of coughs, flatulence, general colds, and fevers. It is ingested as tea or a fermented ginger beer. It is also infused into oils to make a liniment that can help arthritis and other inflammatory conditions because of its strong anti-inflammatory action.

CARIBBEAN PLANT KNOWLEDGE

Modern research has proven that ginger has many compounds that promote healing. It contains capsaicin, which has anti-inflammatory effects. It has enzymes such as zingibain, which dissolves plaque and blood clots and promotes blood and heart health.[20] Because of its antispasmodic effects on smooth muscle, ginger is an effective treatment for menstrual cramps and discomfort.[21]

## Personal Accounts

I have been using ginger in various forms since I was young for cooking and for medicine. As a Caribbean household, we always had ginger in the fridge to cook with or to make tea. I grew it for the first time on my first farm on the Eastern Shore of Maryland; we grew it inside a greenhouse in order to create the right conditions for rhizome growth. Some years, we did not get good rhizomes because we planted it too late in the spring and it needs a longer growing season than most other vegetables in northern climates. In those cases, I would dry the leaves and use them to add flavor to soups and stews as well as to make tea. When I had my daughter, my midwife, Pati Garcia, made me a salve infused with ginger and cannabis to massage on my abdomen to reduce cramping and help everything move back into place. It worked wonders!

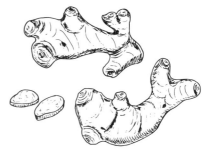

Ginger (*Zingiber officinale*)

---

20  Eugene R. Zampieron, *The Natural Medicine Chest: Natural Medicines to Keep You and Your Family Thriving into the Next Millennium* (M. Evans & Company, 1999).
21  R. Negi et al., "Efficacy of Ginger in the Treatment of Primary Dysmenorrhea: A Systematic Review and Meta-analysis," *Cureus* 13, no. 3 (March 6, 2021): e13743, doi: 10.7759/cureus.13743.

# GUINEA HEN WEED

*Petiveria alliacea*

Common names: gully root, anamu, cudjoe root, mapurite

## Botanical Description

Guinea hen weed has a pungent, garlic-like aroma attributable to the presence of sulfur compounds. The whole plant is used, or the leaves and roots can be used separately. The roots have a stronger smell. The plant is an erect, deeply rooted, vibrant green perennial that grows to a height of about three feet. The stems are thin, and the leaves are alternate, simple, entire, and oblong to elliptic. The flower can be terminal or axillary. The fruit is narrow and oblong with hooks and has a single seed.

## Traditional Knowledge and Modern Research

It is common practice to crush the plant root (which is believed to be more potent than the leaves) and inhale the scent as a treatment for sinusitis. It is often used in herbal baths in Caribbean cultures and Amazon forests. The Garifuna natives in Nicaragua use an infusion or decoction for coughs, cold, pains, and aches and in the performance of specific rituals. Quilombo communities in Brazil prepared a cigarette with it called tira-capeta ("removing the devil"). It is used for anxiety, nervous breakdown, and sleep disturbances.[22]

Guinea hen weed is believed to calm the nerves, control diarrhea, and stimulate the uterus. It is commonly used as an ingredient in women's womb tonics and teas. A tea made from the leaves can be used as nose or eye drops to heal headache, and as nose drops or steam to

---

22    D. A. Luz et al., "Ethnobotany, Phytochemistry and Neuropharmacological Effects of *Petiveria alliacea* L. (Phytolaccaceae): A Review," *Journal of Ethnopharmacology* 185 (June 5, 2016): 182–201, doi: 10.1016/j.jep.2016.02.053.

heal sinusitis. It is used as an analgesic (pain reliever) for muscular pain and to treat skin diseases. It is a common ingredient in bush baths to cure physical and spiritual illness.

Water, methanol, and ethanol extracts of the whole plant have been shown to slow the growth of leukemia cells and several other strains of cancerous tumor cells in vitro. Water extracts of the whole plant have been shown to stimulate the immune system. Root extracts have shown significant anti-inflammatory and pain-relieving effects. Many clinical reports and studies confirm that extracts of the aerial parts and roots have significant broad-spectrum antimicrobial properties against numerous strains of bacteria, viruses, protozoa, fungi, and yeasts.[23]

## Personal Accounts

I tend to make very strong infusions on my first few tries of an herb to get a real feel for the overt and subtle effects. With gully root, I noticed it warmed me, it relaxed me, I almost felt high, and it was a diuretic. I experienced some mild uterine cramping a few hours after I ingested it, and my menstrual cycle came early after three days of drinking a decoction of it consistently. This showed me that it had some reproductive effects and caused me to research that aspect of the plant. I learned that it had been used in Trinidad and other places as a method of abortion. Herbs that were used for abortions usually also doubled as womb cleansers or postpartum tonics.

I didn't have another occasion to use it until 2022. Francis Morean showed it to me growing on the road leading to my house, in preparation for an ethnobotany event called Carnival in The Forest. I harvested it after a rain so that the roots came up easier and intact, and then I dried the whole plant. I began using it in steams whenever my husband had sinusitis, and it helped to clear his sinuses. We even slept

---

23   M. M. Randle et al., "A Systematic Review of the Traditional and Medicinal Uses of *Petiveria alliacea* L. in the Treatment of Chronic Diseases," *Journal of Plant Science and Research* 5, no. 1 (2018): 179–85.

with it by our pillows whenever our toddler was having congestion because just smelling it is powerful! Another anecdote is that when my ninety-three-year-old grandmother was diagnosed with COVID, she lost her sense of smell. The same day she reported losing her smell, I had her steam with gully root, and at the end of the steam session, she told me she could smell again.

# LANI BOIS
*Piper marginatum*
Common names: cake bush, marigold
pepper, ti bombé, anesi wiwiri

## Botanical Description

*Piper marginatum* is a perennial rainforest plant that likes to grow in shady and moist spots. It can be recognized by its unique heart-shaped leaves, which have seven or eight veins running along them, and the strong smell of anise when you crush the leaves. It is native to the Amazon rainforests from South America to the Caribbean. *Marginatum* is part of its Latin name because the stem grows directly out of the leaf margin. It is similar to other members of the Piperaceae family, like *Piper nigrum*, or black pepper, in that the very small flowers grow on a spike that sticks straight up from the leaf margin. Plants of the Piperaceae family with a flower spike are commonly called candlestick bushes in Trinidad.

## Traditional Knowledge and Modern Research

The *Piper* genus of plants has been used in food and medicine throughout the world because its members are native to different continents. In Southeast Asia, people use betel leaf (*Piper betle*). African long pepper (*Piper capense*) is an important traditional medicinal plant. And in South America, lani bois, hoja santa (*Piper auritum*), candle bush (various members of the *Piper* species have this name), and sun hat (*Piper umbellatum*) are different Piperaceae plants that are used traditionally. Lani bois was used by the Indigenous people of the Caribbean, and when Africans and Indians came over, they brought their own traditions based on the ways they used similar plants in their respective countries. In Yoruba culture, *Piper* plants are used in rituals for peace and protection. Plants of this genus have a calming effect on the nervous system and are also routinely used in spiritual baths.

In South America, Indigenous peoples of Colombia call lani bois, curadiente ("teeth cure") because it has analgesic properties and can be stuffed into a tooth cavity for pain relief.[24] Its smell helps repel mosquitoes, so it is crushed and rubbed all over the body as a repellent.

## Personal Accounts

Lani bois grows abundantly in my yard and neighborhood, so I use it often in my bush tea along with other herbs. By itself, I find it has a very calming, sedative effect, so I am careful not to make the tea too strong if I have work to do. I like to use the leaves as a poultice: I chew them up and paste them onto insect bites or small cuts or scrapes to relieve pain, itching, and irritation. Basant, an Indigenous hunter in Trinidad, taught me that lani bois can serve as a deodorant when there is a need to refresh oneself in the bush. He also uses it to enhance his hunting dogs' sense of smell by rubbing it on their noses before a hunt.

---

24  L. G. Sequeda et al., "*Piper marginatum* Jacq. (Piperaceae): Phytochemical, Therapeutic, Botanical Insecticidal and Phytosanitary Uses," *Pharmacology Online* 3 (December 30, 2015): 136–45.

# MANGO LEAF
*Mangifera indica*

## Botanical Description

Mangoes are in the Anacardiaceae family along with famous cousins including cashews, pistachios, and poison ivy. Because of this, some people can have an intense allergic reaction after too much exposure to the skins. *Mangifera indica* can grow to be a very large and old tree. Although it is native to Southeast Asia, it is one of the most common trees on household lots and farms in the Caribbean. It has a short trunk but a wide canopy with leaves that are long, slender, and pointy. There are perhaps hundreds of varieties with different fruit shapes and flavors. Mango trees fruit during the dry season and can flower throughout the year.

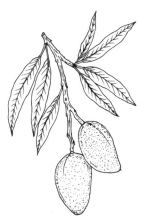

Mangoes
(*Mangifera indica*)

## Traditional Knowledge and Modern Research

Mangoes are one of the most beloved fruits of the Caribbean and around the world. The mango is one of those plants in which every part—flowers, leaves, bark, fruit, and seeds—is considered medicinal and beneficial. The fruits are enjoyed both ripe and unripe. When unripe, they are usually used in chutneys and pickled condiments. They are eaten as a source of vitamin C, vitamin A, and potassium. When the leaves are crushed, they produce a very pleasant scent of turpentine, which is imbued into tea made with them. The tea of young leaves is used for inflammation or virus infection. It is especially used for asthma and arthritis, which are both inflammatory conditions. An elder Rasta told me that it is one of the plants he uses for a chew stick to help with teeth and gums.

## Personal Accounts

One of my favorite sayings about mango came from my cousin Verna McCall, who once noted that mango trees were flowering very abundantly that year. She said her mother used to say, "When mango flowers heavy, hard times are coming." This was another way of saying that God provides. When money is low and it is hard to get groceries, the mango trees will provide the food needed to fill hungry bellies. Two years ago, my father planted a "Julie" mango in my grandmother's yard because every time she eats a mango, she throws the seeds in the yard, hoping they will catch, and now she is delighted to see the tree whenever she looks outside. My great-aunt loves to freeze mango pulp, and my family always joked that when thawed, it is a laxative. I learned firsthand, and now I use frozen mango as a laxative for my daughter when she is constipated.

# NEEM
*Azadirachta indica*

## Botanical Description

Neem is a fast-growing tree in the mahogany (Meliaceae) family that is native to India. It grows in tropical areas around the world where it has been introduced. It has dark green leaves that are compound on the stems and have serrated edges. The leaves create a beautiful and recognizable silhouette in the sky. Its flowers grow in clusters and are beautiful, white, and fragrant. The fruit is considered a drupe and has slightly sweet flesh.

# Traditional Knowledge and Modern Research

Neem has been used in Ayurvedic medicine for thousands of years. It is truly a wonder plant that can be used in medicines, cosmetics, and even agriculture. The leaves are used in the formulation of shampoos and toothpastes, and young twigs can be chewed to help with oral health and for toothbrushing. In the Caribbean especially, neem is used for skin conditions such as eczema and psoriasis because of its antifungal properties. For use on hair, scalp, or skin, it can be applied externally as a wash or soaked into a towel or bandage and placed on the affected areas. It is used for fevers, ear infections, and wound healing because of its anti-inflammatory and antibacterial effects. Finally, the oil from its seeds is well known as an agricultural insecticide.

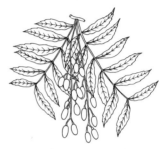

Neem (*Azadirachta indica*)

Neem is used in mosquito repellents and medicines for vector-borne diseases such as malaria and dengue. It is traditionally used in a leaf tea, but it should not be taken for long periods because it can damage the liver and kidneys. Neem is also useful in long-term chronic illnesses such as diabetes and cancer. And research has shown its effectiveness in regulating blood sugar and inhibiting the growth of cancer cells.[25]

---

[25] U. V. Rekha et al., "Known Data on the Therapeutic Use of *Azadiracta indica* (Neem) for Type 2 Diabetes Mellitus," *Bioinformation* 18, no. 2 (February 28, 2022): 82–87, doi: 10.6026/97320630018082.

## Personal Accounts

I first used neem before I ever saw or touched a plant in person. I used it on my organic farm in Maryland as an insecticide and fungicide. The part of the plant used for organic pesticides is the oil from the seed. It disrupts insects' hormones and keeps the insects from molting so that larvae cannot become adults and procreate. It was also effective on our tomatoes when they got fungal blight and our cucurbits when they got powdery mildew.

When I moved to Trinidad, I started to see the tree everywhere! Its leaves and silhouette are very distinctive, and once my mother-in-law showed me the one on their farm, I could easily spot it in other people's yards and land. It has great importance to the Hindu community in Trinidad, so you see it growing in many people's yards for its medicinal and spiritual benefits. In Hindu culture, neem is associated with the goddess Durga and is used to protect and purify a space.

I put neem in a salve that I make for fungal-based eczema and skin issues. I infuse coconut oil and cocoa butter with neem leaves, zebapique, turmeric, wild senna, and cerasee. I also make a tea of the same plants so that it can be taken internally and externally. It is a *very* bitter tea, so people enjoy the topical version much more!

# NONI
*Morinda citrifolia*
Common name: painkiller tree

## Botanical Description

Noni is a small tree in the same family (Rubiaceae) as coffee and ixoras. It is native to the Polynesian islands and was probably brought to the Caribbean in the past few centuries. However, because it grows well through seeds defecated by animals, you can find it growing wild in many places in the Caribbean. The leaves are large and shiny green with prominent veins. The fruit is a compound fruit, like corn. When it is ripe, it has a pungent odor reminiscent of blue cheese.

## Traditional Knowledge and Modern Research

In the Caribbean, noni is traditionally referred to as painkiller tree. The juice from the fruit helps support pain relief and the immune system. The leaves can be made into a tea that supports the immune system, reduces inflammation, and detoxifies the body. It is best to use soft, pale, ripe fruits to make the juice. Fermented noni juice is the traditional way it is used in Polynesia, where it is native. In Guyana, where I learned of the name pain tree, the leaves are crushed in a mortar and pestle and then mixed with coconut oil and rubbed on arthritic joints.

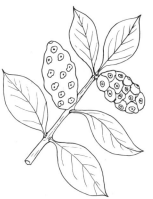

Noni (*Morinda citrifolia*)

Noni is an example of a traditional medicine that has become popular in alternative medicine communities because of exposure on social media. Thousands of memes and graphics tout the healing abilities of this fruit. There have been quite a few studies of noni juice's effects on smokers to see whether it reduced inflammation and oxidative stress. After thirty days of consumption, groups that consumed noni had lower cholesterol levels and reduced free radicals. An extract was given to a group of patients who underwent tooth extraction, and noni reduced pain on par with ibuprofen.[26]

---

26   B. J. West et al., "The Potential Health Benefits of Noni Juice: A Review of Human Intervention Studies," *Foods* 7, no. 4 (April 11, 2018): 58, doi: 10.3390/foods7040058.

## Personal Accounts

My husband spent a couple of years in Polynesia, so he learned from the source about many of the popular Caribbean plants that are native to that region. During his travels in Polynesia, he learned that to make noni juice, a fruit can be placed in an airtight glass container in the sun for a couple of months. During this fermentation, the fruit breaks down and the juice is released. Then the juice is strained out and people take up to one ounce daily. We see noni trees with fruit all the time in our neighborhood and on walks. They are easy to teach children to identify because of their distinctive large, shiny leaves and alien-looking fruit.

# NUTMEG
*Myristica fragrans*

## Botanical Description

Nutmeg is a large evergreen tree that can grow over fifty feet tall. It has shiny green leaves that are oval in shape. Nutmeg is native to Indonesia, and it is popular in the Caribbean as well. The fruit is a drupe, like peaches and nectarines, and it is yellow and splits open when ripe to reveal an oval brown seed with a lacework red covering. It has fragrant yellow flowers that are slightly waxy. The brown seed is a hard kernel that must be cracked open like a nut. Inside is the brain-shaped nutmeg that people grate and use in cooking and medicine. In Trinidad, nutmeg is an important food for the endemic and endangered pawi or piping guan bird.

# Traditional Knowledge and Modern Research

Nutmeg is a beloved spice from Southeast Asia to the Caribbean and everywhere in between. It is one of the common spices used in the Caribbean to flavor teas, punches, porridges, and baked goods. The other spices are cinnamon, bay leaf, allspice, tonka bean, and clove. According to African American traditional midwife Shafia Monroe, it is well known for its warming qualities and is indicated in postpartum care as well as to support healing from colds. Its warming effect is utilized in ointments to soothe aching joints and muscles because nutmeg is a pain reliever and is anti-inflammatory. A pain relief ointment in the Caribbean may have nutmeg, mace, and camphor infused into coconut oil to rub on joints and muscles. A little bit of nutmeg goes a long way, and quantities larger than a tablespoon or so per person have long been known to have hallucinogenic effects, when ingested.

Modern research has shown that nutmeg can lend its psychoactive properties to the compound myristicin, which is similar to MDMA in that it blocks the neurotransmitter acetylcholine. Research also has found that pain reduction is significant in comparison with placebos and other painkillers. One of the most promising areas of use is in

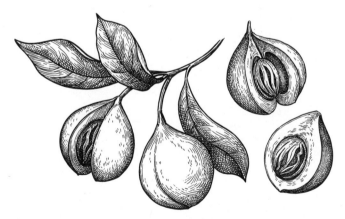

Nutmeg

lowering blood pressure. It works well in its traditional form as a tea or food additive, and it also works well as an extract to isolate specific compounds.[27]

## Personal Accounts

I first encountered nutmeg trees and fruits at a friend's farm in the small village of Montevideo in northeastern Trinidad. Smelling freshly shelled nutmeg versus the powder found in stores blew my mind! The smell is almost intoxicating and keeps drawing you in for more. The red lace covering on the seed has its own special scent profile that is more delicate than the grated seed. It is called mace and is used in baking and herbal medicine preparations.

My husband had an interesting encounter with the wonderful spice. He did not know of its hallucinogenic effects, and one morning while making a smoothie, he made a mistake and shook a container with a few tablespoons of nutmeg into the blender. He did not want to waste it, so he drank it all. He noted that the smoothie was bitter but still palatable. An hour or two later, he began feeling as if he was not on solid ground and could not gauge the distance of objects. He was sweating profusely and very confused because he did not know what was happening. Later that day, as he told me about the smoothie and symptoms, I realized that the nutmeg was the culprit for his weird feelings. He had uncomfortable physical and hallucinatory symptoms for eight to twelve hours as a result of this unintentional "overdose" of nutmeg.

---

27  N. Anripa and V. F. Lone, "Preserving Nutmeg : Historical Significance, Medicinal Benefits, and Climate Change Threats to Indonesian Nutmeg," *International Journal of Islamic and Complementary Medicine* 5, no. 2 (2024): 158–67, doi: 10.55116/ijicm.v5i2.79.

# OKRA
*Abelmoschus esculentus*
Common names: ochro, lady's fingers, gumbo

## Botanical Description

There are wild versions of okra, but the best-known one is planted on farms and in home gardens. It is an annual shrub that grows two to five feet tall and has distinctive lobed leaves. It is a member of the mallow (Malvaceae) family, so its flowers look similar to those of sorrel and cotton. They are pale yellow with a dark red center. The okra fruit is a long, ribbed, fleshy berry that hardens as the seeds mature. The leaves, seeds, and pods are high in mucilage.

## Traditional Knowledge and Modern Research

Okra is indigenous to the African continent, where it has a long tradition in food and medicine. The words "okra" and "gumbo" both come from African words to describe the fruit. Okra is a perfect example of "letting thy food be thy medicine" because of its numerous health benefits. Caribbean cultures rely heavily on okra in dishes such as callaloo and other soups and stews. Pods, leaves, and growing tips may be fried, sauteed, or added to stews. The pods can be dried and

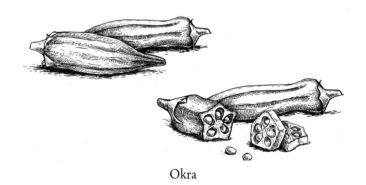

Okra

CARIBBEAN PLANT KNOWLEDGE

ground into powder for soups or sauces, to thicken them and add flavor and nutrients. Okra seeds can be roasted, ground, and used as a caffeine-free coffee substitute.

An elder midwife in Trinidad told me about eating ochroes, as she called them, during the last week of pregnancy to help the baby "slide out." This because of okra's slimy nature, which also makes it good for all mucous membranes, including those of the respiratory and digestive tracts. It helps loosen and release mucus in tissues.

Thanks to recent social media attention, okra has found new life as a health supplement in the form of okra water. People have drunk okra water for ages, but more people have been sharing online about its benefits. In a 2019 study, researchers fed okra water to mice and noted decreases in blood sugar and inflammation in the mice.[28] Although I am happy when trends catch up with traditional knowledge, I think that eating whole okra pods is the best way to enjoy the health benefits. A serving of okra has 13 percent of your daily fiber and 50 percent of daily manganese.[29] Manganese helps the body control blood sugar, and fiber helps with weight loss. This is why okra is also being researched for its antidiabetic and blood sugar–stabilizing effects.

## Personal Accounts

Callaloo is a heartwarming dish that is eaten all around the Caribbean. In some countries, the name applies only to the type of leafy green being used. Depending on the country, and even within a country, "callaloo" can refer to amaranth (*Amaranthus* spp.) or dasheen or taro leaves (*Colocasia esculenta*). It can also just refer to the dish, which

---

28  N. Tyagita et al., "Okra Infusion Water Improving Stress Oxidative and Inflammatory Markers on Hyperglycemic Rats," *Bangladesh Journal of Medical Science* 18, no. 4 (2019): 748–52, doi: 10.3329/bjms.v18i4.42879.

29  A. E. O. Elkhalifa et al., "Okra (*Abelmoschus esculentus*) as a Potential Dietary Medicine with Nutraceutical Importance for Sustainable Health Applications," *Molecules* 26, no. 3 (January 28, 2021): 696, doi: 10.3390/molecules26030696.

may be made with amaranth, dasheen bush, or any other type of bhaji (spinach-type leafy green). I have had callaloo with sweet potato greens, tree spinach, and even Malabar spinach. In Trinidad, the act of making true callaloo always includes coconut milk (fresh is best!) and a copious amount of okra. The slimier, the better!

Callaloo stew is packed with essential vitamins and minerals from greens, pumpkin, okra, coconut milk, onions, garlic, and herbs. It's a great source of dietary fiber and helps you get a few servings of different vegetables in one dish. Eating it regularly and adding lots of healing herbs such as thyme, ginger, garlic, and chadon beni can help reduce inflammation in your body and provide your cells with the fuel they need. My daughter rarely likes eating vegetables alone, but she *loves* callaloo and would eat it daily if she could. Because of her love of this dish, we keep okra and chaya (tree spinach) growing in our yard. We have an almost endless supply of coconuts, and pumpkin is always selling at the vegetable stall, so it is an easy thing to cook for her and feel like she just took a multivitamin!

## Callaloo with Chaya

As I mentioned, callaloo can be made with a variety of different greens, but the key ingredient is okra. I use as much as a pound of okra in my callaloo to ensure we are getting lots of health benefits. For the greens, I like to use chaya, or tree spinach (*Cnidoscolus aconitifolius*), because I have so much of it in my yard and it is always accessible. Chaya is a superfood in its own right and has some of the most micronutrients per gram of any leafy green. It has to be boiled for at least ten to fifteen minutes to evaporate the cyanide compounds in the leaves, rendering it safe to eat. We then put it in the pot with the other callaloo ingredients and cook it down to the desired consistency.

CARIBBEAN PLANT KNOWLEDGE

1–2 pounds chaya leaves (or leaves of amaranth, dasheen, collard, sweet potato, etc.), stems removed, roughly chopped

2 tablespoons oil

2 small onions, chopped

1 small handful broadleaf or fine-leaf thyme

10 garlic cloves, minced

3 pimento peppers, chopped

1 habanero pepper (optional)

½ pound pumpkin, cubed

2 carrots, sliced

1 pound okra, chopped

1 handful chadon beni or cilantro, chopped

2–3 cups coconut milk

salt and black pepper to taste

**Step 1:** Boil the chaya leaves in water for 10–15 minutes and then drain them and set them aside. (If not using chaya, you can skip this step.)

**Step 2:** Place the oil, onions, thyme, garlic, and peppers in a large pot and sauté for 2–3 minutes.

**Step 3:** Add the pumpkin, carrots, and okra and sauté for another minute, and then add the chaya or other greens.

**Step 4:** Add the coconut milk (and water if needed to cover the greens).

**Step 5:** Add the salt and black pepper and bring to a boil.

**Step 6:** Cover and let the callaloo simmer on low heat for 45 minutes to an hour. Stir occasionally. You want to make sure all of the ingredients get soft.

**Step 7:** When everything is cooked and soft, you can use a swizzle stick or an immersion blender to get a smoother consistency or leave it as it is. Some people like it chunky, and some people like it smooth.

**Step 8:** Serve the callaloo hot over rice or with roti, or eat it as a soup.

# PAPAYA
*Carica papaya*
Common name: pawpaw

## Botanical Description

Papaya is a nonwoody tree in the Caricaceae family that is native to South America and the Caribbean. It grows nine to thirty feet tall, depending on cultivation and environment. Its large, bulbous fruit grows directly on the trunk, and its leaves are large, waxy, dark green, and very lobed. Male and female flowers generally grow on separate trees; female flowers are larger. It is a fast-growing and robust tree. The fruit grows at the top of the tree trunk, and you often have to compete with birds and other wildlife for ripe fruit.

## Traditional Knowledge and Modern Research

Every part of the papaya plant has been used for medicine. Most people are familiar with the fruit, which is eaten when pinkish orange and ripe or when light green and unripe. The seeds can be dried and ground to use as a spice similar to black pepper. The fruit and seeds are known for the digestive support they provide. The leaves are considered stronger medicine and are taken in the case of infections that lower a

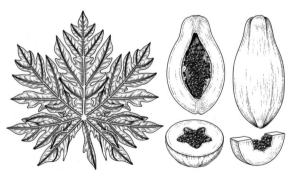

Papaya leaf and fruit

person's blood platelet counts, such as malaria, dengue, and zika. They are bitter, so they are used in blood-building tonics that support the liver and digestion. The caustic white sap from unripe fruits and leaves can be applied to sores and boils to help clear away the dead skin and promote healing. Seeds are eaten for digestive issues and to help expel parasites.

The male pawpaw root is revered highly in traditional medicine. A family friend, Terrence Audain, told us of a venereal disease remedy that used male pawpaw root, charcoal, and molasses to purge the body of the illness and the pathogens that caused it. He saw an elder medicine woman making it one day and asked her what it was and what it was used for.

That conversation with Terrence about the venereal disease remedy started with him telling us that veterinarians in Trinidad were buying up pawpaw leaves from farmers to dry, make into powder, and put into capsules to cure a fever that was spreading among dogs in the country.

Papain is one of the enzymes present in papaya that accounts for some of its medicinal uses. It softens tissues and helps you digest protein from your latest meal, similarly to its modern use as an ingredient in meat tenderizer. It is a common ingredient in digestive health supplements. Because of its use in traditional medicine for viral diseases, it has been studied for use in treating HIV patients. This study showed that a mixture of papaya and guava (*Psidium guajava*) was promising in lowering HIV viral load.[30]

## Personal Accounts

One of my favorite uses of papaya is for my skin care. I like to smash the ripe fruit and paste it on my face. The bromelain in the pulp imme-

---

30  P. Jadaun et al., "Antiviral and ROS Scavenging Potential of *Carica papaya* Linn and *Psidium guajava* Leaves Extract Against HIV-1 Infection," *BMC Complementary Medicine and Therapies* 23, no. 1 (March 18, 2023): 82, doi: 10.1186/s12906-023-03916-x.

diately brightens and tightens skin. I leave it on for fifteen to twenty minutes (pay attention to how your skin reacts and adjust the time accordingly) and then rinse it off and moisturize. I also make a tincture with the fresh leaves that I use in cases of viral or bacterial infections. For dengue, I have juiced the leaves and taken a small shot with lime juice and salt added to cut the bitterness. I would take this shot twice a day for no more than three days and then rest. Papaya is strong medicine and can have strong side effects. An elder once told me that his friend was trying to cure something with papaya leaf juice, drank too much, and got sicker in the other direction! See my essay "Dealing with Dengue" in Chapter 5 for more information about using papaya to treat dengue.

# RATCHETTE

*Opuntia cochenillifera*
Common names: tuna, nopal, cochineal cactus, prickly pear

## Botanical Description

Ratchette is a shrubby succulent plant that can eventually grow hardened stems and reach a height of sixteen feet. Its cactus pads are largely spineless, unlike those of some of its cousins in the *Nopalea* genus. It is an evergreen perennial plant that grows very easily by propagation of the pads, which grow shallow roots easily when placed on soil and will generate new leaf pads quickly. Many different *Opuntia* cactus species are native throughout the Americas, and they look slightly different from *Ratchette* with varying amounts of spikes, pad shapes, and flower colors.

CARIBBEAN PLANT KNOWLEDGE

# Traditional Knowledge and Modern Research

The Latin name of this plant, *Opuntia cochenillifera*, comes from the fact that it is one of the cactus species from which the red dye cochineal was obtained. Spaniards met Indigenous tribes in South America and the Caribbean who knew how to extract the valuable red dye from the insects that this plant hosts. In Trinidad, the pads are cut open and the mucilage inside is used as a shampoo. It is affectionately called Rasta shampoo because it works well to moisturize and cleanse dreadlocked hair. Smaller pads are roasted or heated and placed on any area of pain, swelling, or inflammation as a soothing poultice. The pads are also traditionally prepared as food by boiling, removing the outer layer, and then sautéing them.

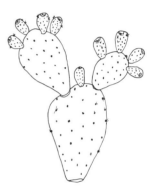

Ratchette (prickly pear)

Research shows that even though there are differences between the domestic and wild versions of *Opuntia* species, they all have high levels of antioxidants and phenols, which are responsible for their nutritional value and medicinal benefits. This is especially helpful when people are suffering from chronic inflammation or stress. They also contain a lot of soluble fiber, pectin, and mucilage, which may help people who suffer from diabetes by slowing the absorption of glucose.[31]

# Personal Accounts

I use this plant as a shampoo at least once a month. It softens my hair and greatly relieves dandruff. My grandmother has multiple ratchette

---

31  M. d. S. S. Díaz et al., "*Opuntia* spp.: Characterization and Benefits in Chronic Diseases," *Oxidative Medicine and Cellular Longevity* (April 9, 2017): 8634249, doi: 10.1155/2017/8634249.

plants growing in her yard, and she mentions that people always ask for a piece to use or propagate. She says that her mother, my great-grandmother, used this plant religiously for everything from medicine to food. It is one of the more widely known plants in Trinidad, and it was one of the first whose uses I learned from my grandmother. I prepare it by slicing a pad in half and scooping out the flesh with a spoon. I then place it in water and use my hands to squeeze and massage the pieces until the water gets thick and viscous. I then strain it, pour it over my hair, lather it in, and rinse it out.

# SANTA MARIA

*Lippia alba*

Common names: colic mint, bushy lippia

## Botanical Description

Santa Maria is in the verbena family, Verbenaceae. It can grow to four or five feet tall, with sprawling bushy, woody stems. The light green, serrated, and textured leaves grow opposite the branches, with tiny flowers that bud at intersections. It is a favorite flower of many pollinators; when it is flowering, there is constant action around the plant. It grows very well from cuttings, and it can endure clay soil and some drought. The leaves when crushed have a pleasant minty, musky scent. There are at least two varieties of this species. One has more of a minty smell, and the other has more of a citrus smell.

## Traditional Knowledge and Modern Research

In Jamaica, Santa Maria is known as colic mint. It is given for stomach ailments and gripes (intestinal pain), hence the name. It is known to reduce gas and soothe the gastrointestinal tract. It can help relieve menstrual pain, especially when mixed with ginger. It is a common ingredient in herbal bush baths and can help with fever when used in a bath. Santa Maria also can be made into syrup for coughs and respiratory issues. It is known as a safe, effective, and regularly used bush medicine. In Trinidad and Tobago, one of the common names is twa tas, which is French creole for "three cups." This alludes to the fact that it tastes so good, you can never drink only one cup! It is a favorite bedtime tea for children in Caribbean households.

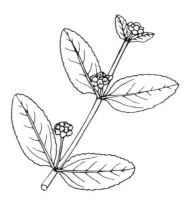

Santa maria *(Lippia alba)*

Modern research has shown that the effectiveness of fragrant plants like this one comes from the essential oils they release. Essential oils are the parts of the plant that confer benefits like antibacterial, antifungal and antiviral effects. The essential oils in *Lippia alba* contain two main constituents, citral (an aldehyde) and limonene (a terpene). The reason why *Lippia alba* soothes the digestive, respiratory, and reproductive organs is that its essential oils have antispasmodic properties.[32]

## Personal Accounts

This is one of my go-to bush teas for myself and my family. My daughter diligently goes to harvest some when she is feeling the need for bush tea and brings me a cup with leaves in it to pour hot water over. I fell in love with it while I was pregnant and noticed that it almost instantly relieved my heartburn and acid reflux. My daughter was born with a head full of thick hair, and they say that contributes to heartburn during pregnancy, so I had my fair share! I would pour boiling water

---

32   P. M. M. Carvalho et al., "Effect of the *Lippia alba* (Mill.) N.E. Brown Essential Oil and Its Main Constituents, Citral and Limonene, on the Tracheal Smooth Muscle of Rats," *Biotechnology Reports* 17 (March 2018): 31–34, doi: 10.1016/j.btre.2017.12.002.

over five to seven leaves in a cup and let it steep. The smell alone helped to soothe my digestive system. The essential oils create an overall sense of well-being when the tea is drunk, and it gives mental clarity. When I have respiratory issues, I add Santa Maria to a pot of hot water with Spanish thyme (*Plectranthus amboinicus*) and gully root (*Petiveria alliacea*) for sinus relief.

# SERIYO
*Sambucus simpsonii*
Common names: elderflower, elderberry

## Botanical Description

This is a shrub that grows up to twenty feet in height. It has serrated leaves that are oppositely arranged. The flowers are small, white, and fragrant and grow in abundance in large clusters. The fruit is black or purplish black. This species does not fruit as often in the Caribbean as it does in other climates. It is closely related to, and looks just like, common American elderberry (*Sambucus canadensis*).

## Traditional Knowledge and Modern Research

Although most cultures know the leaves to be poisonous, they are used for their purgative property in the Caribbean. Elders say to juice the leaves or drink a tea made of them to purge the system. The flowers are used for coughs and colds and to bring down fevers. The flowers are traditionally made into a syrup, alone or combined with other herbs that act on the respiratory system, such as carpenter grass (*Justicia pectoralis*) or kooze mahoe (*Urena lobata*). The juice of the leaves is especially indicated for asthma. It is said to drink a shot of the juice in the morning and evening for seven days. On the third or fourth day, you will be nauseated and may throw up, but by the seventh day you will feel better.

The elderflower/elderberry plant has been well studied. The berries are the most famous part of the plant, and they are ingested in a syrup or a tea or raw to boost the immune system and reduce fever. Elderberry is a widely available supplement in over-the-counter medicines and is touted for its immune-boosting abilities.

## Personal Accounts

I first encountered seriyo growing in the yard of a midwife named Miss Alice Prentice in Barrackpore (see her interview in Chapter 5), Trinidad. She told me she used the leaves to treat asthma. I was surprised to see it, as I didn't think elderberry grew in Trinidad. While farming in Maryland, I grew American elderberry shrubs. I was told by friends at Perennial Roots Farm on the Eastern Shore of Virginia that these plants are truly the elders on the farm and can create a network or sharing between plants at the root and mycelial level. From experience, they noted that planting elderberry along the borders of fields made better soil and harvests.

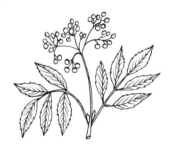

Seriyo

I later learned that is the same genus but a different species and that the flowers and leaves have similar constituents to the elderberry I grew up seeing in Maryland, growing wild and cultivated. I then saw a shrub growing in my neighborhood that I was able to get cuttings from and start growing at home. From growing it and observing it here in Trinidad, I have not seen any berries form. This could be because of a lack of specific pollinators or the type of cultivars.

I soak the flowers in puncheon rum to create a tincture, which I use to boost my immune system before and during travel or at the first sign of sickness.

# SHANDILAY
*Leonotis nepetifolia*
Common names: man piaba, lion bush, cough bush,
klip dagga, lions ear, Christmas candlestick

## Botanical Description

Shandilay is native to Africa but is also common in South America and the Caribbean. This plant is in the Lamiaceae family, along with herbs such as mint, basil, rosemary, and sage. One identifying characteristic of this family is the square stems on most plants. The plants are also full of aromatic compounds that translate into healing powers. Shandilay is loosely branched, with thick square green stems. The leaves are wide and in opposite pairs along the stem. The rounded flower heads develop in small, spiny clusters that encircle the stem. The spikes of each spiny cluster will open up, allowing orange petals to emerge; some say they look like a lion's ear, which gave the plant one of its common names. It can be cultivated, but all the ones in my yard have voluntarily grown. It will quickly take over an area because of the abundance of small seeds dispersed from each plant. They seem to love water and rich soil, and they take off and grow fast once the rainy season starts.

## Traditional Knowledge and Modern Research

Shandilay got the name dagga, which is another name for cannabis, because in some cultures it is dried and smoked and causes a mild euphoric effect. In Trinidad, it is used widely as a treatment for fever, coughs, colds, asthma, and diabetes. It is either made into a tea or pounded and juiced. The flavor of the tea and pure juice is very bitter, but often the best medicines are bitter! The juice can be cut with salt to make it more palatable. One of the common names in Guyana is man piaba. This speaks to traditional knowledge that it is a plant more for men than for women. An elder parang singer from Moruga, Trinidad, once told me that women really should not drink too much of this tea.

Leonurine is the active constituent of shandilay. It is an alkaloid that has demonstrated antidepressant-like effects and has been shown to increase levels of serotonin, noradrenaline, and dopamine. This accounts for its relaxing and psychoactive effects. Researchers noted that "the therapeutic power of *L. nepetifolia* has been attributed to its phytochemical contents, including alkaloids, tannins, saponins, flavonoids, steroids, and terpenoids. Several studies have confirmed that these phytochemicals protect humans against disease-causing organisms."[33]

## Personal Accounts

Shandilay bush is always growing in my Great-Aunty Doris's yard in South Oropouche, Trinidad. She calls it shandilay or cough bush, and she was the first to tell me about its uses to support colds and coughs. I mix a few leaves in with other plants, like lemongrass (*Cymbopogon citratus*), Spanish thyme (*Plectranthus amboinicus*), and Santa Maria (*Lippia alba*), to make a tea. A woman on the Eastern Shore of Maryland told me that she used to grow a version of this plant (*Leonotis leonurus*) for her husband as a marijuana replacement.

---

[33] R. Gang and Y. Kang, "Botanical Features and Ethnopharmacological Potential of *Leonotis nepetifolia* (L.) R. Br: A Review," *Journal of Plant Biotechnology* 49, no. 1 (2022): 3–14, doi: 10.5010/JPB.2022.49.1.003.

# SORREL

*Hibiscus sabdariffa*

Common names: roselle, flor de Jamaica

## Botanical Description

Sorrel is a flowering plant in the Malvaceae (mallow) family of plants, which also includes cacao, okra, and cotton. Its leaves are lobed, with three to five fingers, and it can grow up to seven feet tall. It has pale yellow flowers with dark red in the center. The fleshy, dark red calyx is the most-used part of the plant. It is a drought-tolerant plant, and the calyxes usually form and are harvested in the dry season. The hibiscus family has hundreds of species native to Africa and Asia. You will note Hibiscus *rosa-sinensis* flowers accompanying the numbers at the bottom of the pages of this book.

## Traditional Knowledge and Modern Research

Sorrel calyxes are usually steeped to make tea and refreshing drinks, and the leaves are cooked as a nutritional green in soups and stews. The leaves can also be eaten raw and make a great addition to salads. Sorrel is considered cooling, moistening, and astringent and is used as a tea or vaginal steam for women to tone and rejuvenate the uterus and vagina, especially during pregnancy and postpartum. A 2023 article in a scientific journal noted, "Calyces formulations are used in Egypt to treat heart and nervous system disorders, promote urination, and act as a cooling agent. Calyces of *H. sabdariffa* are used in Sudan to treat high blood pressure, cold symptoms, and flu."[34] Similar to okra seeds, sorrel seeds have traditionally been used as a stimulant coffee

---

34    O. B. Onyeukwu et al., "*Hibiscus sabdariffa*—Uses, Nutritional and Therapeutic Benefits—A Review," *Journal of Bioscience and Biotechnology Discovery* 8, no. 2 (2023): 18–23, doi: 10.31248/jbbd2023.178.

CARIBBEAN PLANT KNOWLEDGE

substitute. In the Caribbean, sorrel is usually ready to harvest around Christmas, so it is mixed with spices, ginger, and sugar and enjoyed as a favorite holiday drink.

Plants that are steeped in tradition usually have many other benefits besides taste, and the traditions evolved with humans to help us survive. Our ancestors understood sorrel to be nutritious, but modern research has shown that it has high amounts of vitamin C, calcium, iron, riboflavin, niacin, and antioxidant compounds.[35] The red color is due to anthocyanin compounds, which are responsible for many of its medicinal benefits.

## Personal Accounts

I grew up with sorrel as a Christmas treat. There was always a bag of dried sorrel in the pantry that got taken out on Christmas Eve to make a strong sorrel drink that I loved. Everyone prepares sorrel slightly differently, and at this point I can tell if someone in my family or my husband's family made the sorrel with my eyes closed! The following is a general recipe that can be changed and adapted based on ingredients in your pantry and your taste buds. As I have more access in Trinidad to fresh and dried sorrel, I drink it often as a simple tea without sugar. With the leftover calyxes from making tea, I make jams and chutneys with sugar and spices. Sorrel is also fun to use in natural dye experiments with my daughter. Similarly to St. John's bush, its dye bath color can change depending on pH.

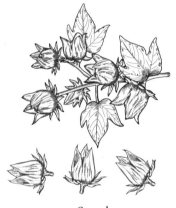

Sorrel

---

35  Onyeukwu et al., "*Hibiscus sabdariffa*."

CARIBBEAN HERBALISM

## Sorrel

To make jam after making this tea, you can boil down the remnants of the sorrel with 2 parts sorrel to 1 part sorrel water or lime juice to 1 part sugar. Adjust the sugar to your liking. To make chutney, simmer the sorrel remnants with herbs (e.g., chadon beni, ginger, garlic) and spices (e.g., geera, cumin, curry leaf). I like to sneak medicinal plants like wonder of the world (*Kalanchoe pinnata*) into sauces and chutneys that already have bitter and tart flavors because the flavors hide well in the strong chutney.

1 pound fresh sorrel
6 cups water
4 West Indian bay leaves
(*Pimenta racemosa*)
1½ cinnamon sticks
2 small pinches
dried clove

1 half-inch piece
ginger, cleaned and
sliced or diced
1 orange peel
a few dashes
Angostura bitters
sugar or sweetener
to taste

**Step 1:** Separate the sorrel sepals from the seed pods. Visually inspect sorrel for any defective pieces.

**Step 2:** In a large pot, bring the water to a boil and add everything except the sorrel.

**Step 3:** Once the water is boiling again, bring it down to a simmer and add the sorrel. Stir well and let the mixture simmer, covered, for 20 minutes.

**Step 4:** Remove the pot from the heat and let the infusion steep for at least 2 hours but preferably overnight.

**Step 5:** Strain out the sorrel and spices. Set them aside for potential reuse in a weaker batch or in jam or chutney.

**Step 6:** Add the sugar or sweetener of choice and the Angostura bitters to taste.

**Step 7:** Bottle the infusion and let it "age" for a couple of days on the counter before refrigerating.

# SOURSOP
*Annona muricata*
Common names: graviola, guanabana

## Botanical Description

Soursop is an evergreen tree native to the tropical Americas, but it is now found in tropical regions around the world. It has broad leaves and large green oblong heart-shaped fruits that are covered with soft green spikes. The inside of the fruit contains a white pulp with black seeds, which is extremely fragrant and has a strong flavor and custard-like texture. It is in the Annonaceae family, also known as the custard apple family. The fruit is picked before it fully ripens and falls to the ground.

## Traditional Knowledge and Modern Research

The fruit of the tree is eaten when ripe, and in traditional medicine a leaf tea is ingested. The leaf tea is considered cooling and is used to treat high blood pressure, expel parasites, and treat insomnia. The smell of the soursop leaf is considered a sedative; leaves can be crushed and placed on a pillow for insomnia. In Trinidad, according to Sylvia Moodie-Klubalsingh's book *Maljo, Bush Teas and Secret Prayers*, a tea of soursop leaf mixed with West Indian bay leaf (*Pimenta racemosa*) is prepared for people who have nausea or

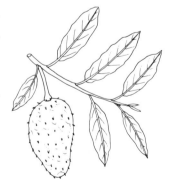

Soursop

feel generally unwell.[36] Since ancient times, it has been used as a food crop as well as a medicine. According to Francis Morean, in Tobago the unripe fruits are soaked in water and then the infused water is used as a blood cleanser or tonic.

Today, soursop health supplements are very popular in the form of tea, pills, and powders. The fruit pulp can also be found around the world in international grocery section freezers, and it is a popular addition to ice cream, smoothies, and drinks. According to a scientific review of different studies of soursop, all parts of the tree exhibit anti-cancer activity. Scientists tested soursop extracts on cell lines of different cancers and noted antigrowth activity on tumors and increased cell death in cancer cells.[37] This is called an in vitro study, meaning in the lab, whereas tests on humans or animals would be considered in vivo. When reading modern research, it is important to note whether the results come from in vitro or in vivo studies.

## Personal Accounts

I have a soursop tree growing along my driveway. It fruits occasionally, but we rarely can harvest because the fruit is a favorite of ants, which will devour a small fruit before it is ripe enough to pick. However, the leaves are always abundant. The first time I used the leaf for medicine was while I was lactating to help increase my milk supply, along with blue vervine. My mother suffers from insomnia, so when she was visiting, I created a tea for her that included soursop leaves, blue vervine, and passion fruit leaves. She loved it. Now, whenever I visit her in Baltimore, I bring leaves for her to make her own tea. She once told me that crushing and smelling the leaves alone brought relaxation

---

36    Sylvia Moodie-Kublalsingh, *Maljo, Bush Teas and Secret Prayers: Trinidad Cocoa Panyols' Beliefs* (Greentree Press, 2021).

37    A. K. Qazi et al., "Emerging Therapeutic Potential of Graviola and Its Constituents in Cancers," *Carcinogenesis* 39, no. 4 (February 15, 2018): 522–33, doi: 10.1093/carcin/bgy024.

to her mind and calmed her spirit, so I always recommend that she crush some leaves and put them in her pillowcase.

# SPANISH NEEDLE
*Bidens alba, B. pilosa*
Common names: railway daisy, needle grass, beggar-ticks

## Botanical Description

*Bidens pilosa* is an annual erect herbaceous plant that is native to South America but has spread all over the world. It is a member of the Asteraceae family. It has lobed and serrated leaves that form opposite of each other. The flowers are white with a yellow center, and the seeds are long and narrow spikes (hence the name needle grass) that stick to clothing and fur for dispersal through an ecosystem. They grow well in disturbed soils along roadways and railways, on farms, and in urban environments.

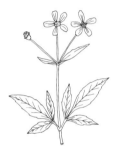

Spanish needle

## Traditional Knowledge and Modern Research

The entire plant is edible and medicinal. The flower makes a tangy addition to salads. Shoots, tips, and young leaves are good for adding nutrients to your soup or sautéed veggies. Railway daisy tastes like spinach. The leaves make a hearty tea full of vitamin C and iron. The dried leaves can be infused into oils to make nourishing salves and balms or soaps that heal the skin. It is especially indicated for viral and bacterial conditions that cause inflammation in our bodies. It is also known to help strengthen the immune system.

Railway daisy's long taproot is a bio accumulator of heavy metals, so it can be used to remediate the effects of heavy metal in soils. This also means you may want to approach *Bidens* species growing in industrial sites or known lead or cadmium hot spots with caution. Its extracts are also used in beauty products for their retinol-like effect on skin. It is an amazing source of plant-based retinol.

## Personal Accounts

I have used the tincture of this herb as a preventive measure against cold and flu. A person that I gifted a bottle reported that the tincture helped ease their allergy-induced sinus issues. I make poultices of it to put on areas of inflammation such as bug bites, or even mastitis when I was breastfeeding. It is a great first aid tool. When I need a boost of iron, I drink tea made from this plant. *Bidens* is very nutritious, and I try to use a little of it in my food or as a tea at least once a week.

# SPANISH THYME

*Coleus amboinicus*
Common names: Cuban oregano, big leaf thyme,
podina, Indian borage, Mexican mint

## Botanical Description

This herb possibly originated in Africa and India, but is widespread across the continents. It is straggly and thick-stemmed, with fuzzy leaves that are in opposite pairs along the stem and are broad with tapered tips. It is semi-succulent and has a strong oregano/thyme odor with hints of turpentine. Pale purple flowers are arranged in clusters at the tips of branches.

# Traditional Knowledge and Modern Research

From Africa and India, this plant made its way to Europe and then over to the Americas via Spanish traders (hence the name Spanish thyme). Its most common use in the Caribbean, and especially Trinidad, is as a component of green seasoning, which is a fragrant and delicious mix of chadon beni, pimento peppers, garlic, onions, and ginger, with Spanish thyme as the star. Therefore, it is a regular part of every Trinidadian's diet. The leaves can be heated and placed across the nose or head for sinusitis or headache. A tea or decoction of the leaves is used for stomach, sinus, and respiratory issues.

The essential oil content of this plant is of modern interest because it is high in thymol, a strong antiviral agent. Thymol is a major ingredient in cleaners that are approved for organic use on food surfaces.

# Personal Accounts

Spanish thyme is probably one of the first herbs I could name and recognize because it was used all the time in my father's Trinidadian cooking at home. Even though I grew up in Baltimore, Maryland, outside of its normal habitat, my father always had a plant growing indoors that he picked to cook and make green seasoning. My family never used it as medicine when I was growing up, but I started drinking it as a tea when I moved to Trinidad, where I have a large patch growing in my yard. It grows so abundantly that it begs you to use it. My daughter picks it for herself whenever she wants some "bush tea" and brings it to me to make a cup for her. It has a soothing minty flavor with some bitter undertones. I use it as a safe general-use tea but also acutely when feeling cough or cold symptoms arising. I have found that the flavor and constituents preserve well in glycerin extractions and in syrup. So I will soak it with cough bush (*Leonotis nepetifolia*) and Santa Maria (*Lippia alba*) in glycerin and use it as a cough medicine. Alternatively, I have made a lovely cough syrup by reducing Spanish thyme with sorrel (*Hibiscus sabdariffa*) and sugar or honey.

# ST. JOHN'S BUSH
*Justicia secunda, Dianthera secunda*
Common names: blood root, sanguinaria

## Botanical Description

St. John's bush is an herbaceous plant that is native to South America and the Caribbean but is also grown in Africa for medicinal purposes. It is evergreen and perennial, with a sturdy stem that can sometimes become woody. The leaves are opposite, glossy, and oval shaped. The flowers are a dark pinkish red and are one of the signature ways to identify the plant, based on their tube shape. It grows along rivers, streams, and gullies and is a favorite of long-billed hummingbirds because of the flower shape.

## Traditional Knowledge and Modern Research

This plant is used in Trinidad as a bush bath for babies and adults to help with skin conditions and for spiritual protection. In West Africa, it has been planted as an ornamental but also used as a tea to help with anemia. When you crush the leaves and make tea, the water turns a dark reddish purple. Traditional healers would have seen this and, knowing the doctrine of signatures, immediately attributed it to a positive action on blood. It is also used to treat menstrual disorders and to replenish iron after menstruation. It can also be steamed and eaten as an addition to soups or stews.

A few studies have shown the presence of bioactive healing compounds such as tannins, flavonoids, alkaloids, and anthocy-

CARIBBEAN PLANT KNOWLEDGE

anins (which, similarly to their presence in red cabbage, cause the color change in water). It has also been found to have high levels of bioavailable iron, which speaks to its use as a treatment for anemia. According to a paper from a Nigerian university, *Justicia secunda* has high levels of iron, calcium, selenium, and other minerals. In tests on mice, it significantly raised hemoglobin and platelet numbers in test subjects, which corroborates traditional wisdom.[38]

## Personal Accounts

This plant grows all around my neighborhood in Trinidad. I first heard about it from a friend, Shalizahr Belgrove, who said she used it as a spiritual plant in protection rituals. It is not to be mistaken with St. John's wort, but they most likely share part of a name because they both turn water red. I started using it when I was in my third trimester of pregnancy to help raise my hematocrit numbers until my midwife was satisfied that I was not too anemic to have a home birth. It truly worked! It tastes like a hearty spinach and makes a good potherb to put in soups or stews. I also have experimented with making natural fabric dyes out of the reddish-purple decoction of leaves. Because of the presence of tannins and anthocyanins, its color does lend itself to fabric beautifully, but the dye fades pretty fast. The colors ranged from purple to green, depending on the pH of the dye bath. I was able to change the color of the dye bath by adding fresh lemon juice (acidic and pink tones) or baking soda (basic and blue-green tones) to change the acidity to the desired level of color. Because of this, St. John's bush can act as a pH indicator for other substances.

---

38   C. R. Onyema et al., "Haematological and Biochemical Studies on *Justicia secunda* Infusion Used in Treatment of Anaemia," *GSC Advanced Research and Reviews* 20, no. 2 (2024): 57–68, doi: 10.30574/gscarr.2024.20.2.0286.

# TI-MARIE

*Mimosa pudica*

Common names: shame bush, sensitive plant, touch-me-not

## Botanical Description

Ti-Marie is native to Central and South America but can now be found all over the world. It is a member of the pea family, Fabaceae. It grows in disturbed soils, on abandoned lots, and on farmland as an abundant weed, which can be hard to remove by hand because of the tiny thorns along its stem. It is a creeping shrub with small green leaves that close when touched or at night. Its bright pink to purple flowers look like puff balls. The roots go deep into the soil to collect nutrients, and they repair the soil as a result of their nitrogen-fixing ability.

## Traditional Knowledge and Modern Research

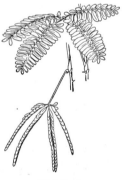

Ti-Marie

This is one of the most well-known and easily identified Caribbean herbs because every child remembers the joy of passing through a field of them and making them close with a light brush of a finger. The root is the most potent part of the plant, and it can be collected and prepared as a tea. Most people use it for kidney, urinary, and menstrual issues. In the Caribbean, kidney issues are usually called "stoppage of water," and this plant is indicated for urinary blockages. The roots of the plant are pounded or chewed into a poultice to put on snakebites or scorpion stings. The leaves can be pounded into a poultice for skin issues or boiled and drunk as a tea.

## Personal Accounts

I first encountered ti-Marie as a young child in my grandmother's yard in Trinidad. It grew between her gate and the road, on a thin strip of pavement that was inadvertently home to many different medicines that are also considered "weeds." Roadsides are often living apothecaries for the diversity in plant life thanks to the movement of wind and to the human and animal excrements that deposit seeds along these popular pathways. Ti-Marie is considered a pesky weed by many gardeners and a medicinal treasure chest by traditional herbalists. I realized the wide range of this plant when visiting Thomas Jefferson's Monticello plantation in Virginia, where a labeled patch of this plant was growing in the garden.

# TURMERIC
*Curcuma longa*
Common names: saffron, haldi

## Botanical Description

Turmeric is the orange tuberous rhizome of an herbaceous plant in the Zingiberaceae (ginger) family. It is originally from Southeast Asia but has traveled around the world. It grows well in most tropical areas and can be grown in temperate regions in greenhouses or in modified microclimates. The mature rhizomes are brown on the outside and dark orange on the inside, whereas the immature ones are pale orange inside. Although it flowers, it does not have seeds, so when it is being cultivated, some rhizomes are left in the ground or collected to propagate and continue the crop. It is usually planted in the beginning of the rainy season and ready to harvest during the dry season, when the green leaves die back and more energy is sent to the rhizomes.

# Traditional Knowledge and Modern Research

Turmeric has been used as a food, dye, and medicine for many centuries. It is a staple of Southeast Asian and Caribbean cooking and has long been known to decrease inflammation in the body, especially from arthritis. It is also known to calm the stomach for people with indigestion. Turmeric has been used in Ayurveda and traditional Chinese medicine, which made their way to the Caribbean via immigrants. Because of its yellow color, the doctrine of signatures would have shown practitioners in the past that it was good for jaundice (yellowing of skin and eyes) due to liver illness. So it has also traditionally been used to support the liver and cleanse the blood. It is most often drunk as a tea in the morning with a little coconut milk or cow's milk to make a golden milk tea. The dried powder or fresh root is also made into a paste that can be rubbed on blemishes or areas of arthritic pain. Traditionally, it has been known that the effects of turmeric are heightened when black pepper and fat or oil are added to the preparation.

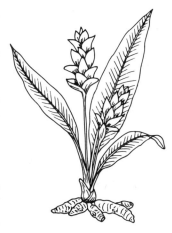

Turmeric

Turmeric is a traditional plant medicine that has been studied extensively, and modern research comes to the same conclusions as traditional knowledge. Curcumin has been found to be the main active component, and it is considered a polyphenol. In modern times, curcumin is extracted from the turmeric plant and included in arthritis creams. When researchers administered 1,200 milligrams per day of curcumin and compared it with cortisone, curcumin was found to work better orally than the powerful pain drug for relieving inflammation, without any side effects.[39] The dye is also a very common ingredient used in foods to impart a yellow-orange color.

## Personal Accounts

Turmeric has been in my kitchen cabinet my whole life. Having Trinidadian roots and growing up in the United States meant turmeric was used often in our dishes, such as split pea dal or curries. My Great-Aunt Doris swears by the turmeric and coconut milk tea she drinks every morning, and I can attest that for a woman in her eighties, she is extremely strong and healthy. Thanks to my husband's foresight many years ago, we have a large patch of turmeric growing that gets larger every year, and we harvest whenever we need it for spices or medicine. When I plan to powder the rhizomes, I first blanch them in boiling water for twenty minutes and then set them out to dry. This breaks down some of the starches and makes them easier to dry and powder. With fresh roots, I make either a tea or a tincture (by soaking in alcohol with black pepper for four weeks) to take whenever I have a cold or other inflammatory condition.

When the green vegetative part aboveground dies down during the dry season, around December–January every year, is considered the best time to harvest. However, you can get a small harvest at any time of year. My mother-in-law, Gloria Parris, was the first person to tell me that you should use oil and black pepper with turmeric in order to unlock its healing powers. She uses it for her arthritis. She is of East Indian heritage, so she holds many generations of turmeric use in her bones.

---

39  Eugene R. Zampieron, *The Natural Medicine Chest: Natural Medicines to Keep You and Your Family Thriving into the Next Millennium* (M. Evans & Company, 1999).

# WONDER OF THE WORLD
*Kalanchoe pinnata*
Common names: leaf of life, mother of thousands, miracle leaf

## Botanical Description

*Kalanchoe* is a genus in the Crassulaceae family. This family mainly originated in Madagascar, though different species of *Kalanchoe* have made it to the Caribbean. Kalanchoe is a succulent plant with opposite leaves that have serrated edges. The flowers are pendulous and pink and look like bells. The plant grows low to the ground and can tolerate many adverse conditions including drought and shade, thanks to its ability to store water and prevent it from evaporating. There are many species in the *Kalanchoe* genus, and although they differ, they are often given the same names because of similar properties. The mother of thousands name comes from the way it propagates itself by forming "baby plants" and/or roots on the leaf margins, which drop to the ground and produce a mature plant.

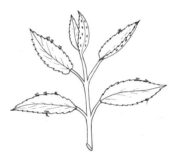

Kalanchoe pinnata

## Traditional Knowledge and Modern Research

This plant received names like wonder of the world, leaf of life, and miracle leaf because of its remarkable healing ability. Although all parts of the plant are medicinal, the most-used part is the leaf juice. This is extracted through squeezing, chewing, blending, pounding, or heating. Heating a leaf until it is slightly translucent and then placing it on a bruise or sore can greatly help with inflammation and wound healing. A tea made of the leaves or an extraction of the leaf juice is used to treat bronchitis and other respiratory issues.

## Personal Accounts

A version of kalanchoe that is more often called mother of thousands than wonder of the world grows all over my grandmother's yard. I remember coming to Trinidad when I was younger and being told to chew it up and put it on my bug bites to help with the swelling and itching, along with aloe vera. Over twenty years later, I was able to use the plant to help my grandmother heal some internal bruising after she fell and hurt her eye. I heated a leaf over a fire and let it cool before placing it on her bruise. It works well as a bandage, and you can add other treatments, such as castor oil, under the leaf. It has a slightly bitter flavor, but I enjoy eating a leaf when I am working outside. A good remedy for a cold is to heat a few leaves over a fire and then squeeze the juice into a container. You may get one or two tablespoons of juice, to which you can add honey and lime and take as a shot twice a day while symptoms persist.

# ZEBAPIQUE
*Neurolaena lobata*
Common names: jackass bitters, tres puntas

*"But let's say you have a serious cold, you get a virus. It have you mash up. I have ah mixture there. It very, very good. You see the Zeb-a-pik . . . Zeb-a-pik . . . Cudjoe root. Mash up both of them. Boil them very strong. Strain it properly. Use a cloth. Not strainer. Add puncheon rum and*

*Noilly Pratt vermouth. Grind clove. If you know people does come here for that mixture. Throw it in the throat."*

Leo Telesford, as interviewed by Francis Morean, October 1998

## Botanical Description

*Neurolaena lobata* grows in margins of the rainforest and areas of human civilization and in disturbed sites such as roadsides and fields. It is a member of the Asteraceae family and is native to the Caribbean and Central America. It has slender dark green leaves that have three lobes when they are mature. It has small yellow flowers that bloom toward the end of the rainy season, which make it an excellent addition to a pollinator garden. It is an extremely bitter plant; hence its common name jackass bitters.

## Traditional Knowledge and Modern Research

This plant is well loved across the Caribbean and South America. It can be infused into water, alcohol, or honey, or its leaves can be crushed and juiced. The juiced liquid can be rubbed on infected skin to heal rashes and minor wounds. The bitter liquid is considered a cure-all for acute illnesses such as colds, coughs, infections, parasites, and fevers. It is also recommended for long-term ailments like diabetes. It helps regulate glucose levels. The bitter constituent is a blood builder and tonic. It is a common ingredient in multiherbal formulations. You will often find it on shelves in Caribbean households preserved in rum or wine (alone or with other roots and herbs). People will take a small shot of this at the first sign of illness. It is traditionally used in moderation, and only a few leaves are boiled to make a strong tea that can be taken throughout the day.

Research has supported its traditional uses. The journal *Phytochemistry* published an article in 2013 about the anti-inflammatory effects of zebapique due to the presence of sesquiterpene lactones, which are known to reduce inflammation in the body caused by colds, infections, and wounds.[40]

## Personal Accounts

Zebapique is perhaps one of the most famous remedies in Trinidad and Tobago. Although the plant grows wild, sometimes it is cultivated in home gardens for ease of use. "Zeb" means "herb" in French, and "pique" means "bitter." We cultivate this herb on our land and it is found growing on our friends farms and river banks in our neighborhood. I make a tincture of the herb in puncheon rum to preserve its medicinal qualities. I take this tincture at the first sign of flu or fever. When I have access to fresh leaves, I dry them and also make herbal teas when I have an illness. I usually only add half a leaf of zebapique to about 2 cups of water and drink it throughout the day. It is VERY potent! Within minutes of drinking some of the tea, I can feel fever and flu symptoms subside in my body, thanks to the powerful anti-inflammatory compounds in this plant. It is also one of my favorite herbs to include in preparations for the skin. I make a zebapique herbal oil by infusing it into coconut oil by itself or with herbs like comfrey and cerasee. Then I add cocoa butter and beeswax to make a healing salve to place on eczema patches or bug bites.

---

40   B. Walshe-Roussel et al., "Potent Anti-inflammatory Activity of Sesquiterpene Lactones from *Neurolaena lobata* (L.) R. Br. ex Cass., a Q'eqchi' Maya Traditional Medicine," *Phytochemistry* 92 (August 2013): 122–27, doi: 10.1016/j.phytochem.2013.05.004.

# SOME ADDITIONAL PLANTS

**Cerasee or Caraili (*Momordica charantia*)**

This is a vine in the Cucurbitaceae family that grows wild in the Caribbean along fences and roadsides everywhere. The wild version has a much smaller fruit than the bitter melon bought in stores. It is used as a cooling cleanse that is taken for colds, diabetes, and high blood pressure. According to Gloria Parris, it is one of the best herbs to drink to help with menstrual pain.

**Cotton (*Gossypium* spp.)**

According to a healer named Raymond Julien in Gasparillo village in Santa Cruz, Trinidad, mothers should use this on babies under six months of age to clean out their system and make them healthy for life. He said that if you give children this as a diluted tea when they are a few months old, they will never have skin issues in the future.

**Ditay Payee (*Capraria biflora*)**

This is a very common herb in the Caribbean that is well known as an eye medicine to treat inflammation or conjunctivitis. It aids in overall maintenance of eyes and prevention of eye diseases and is considered cooling. I make a tea of the leaves and when it cools, I soak two cotton

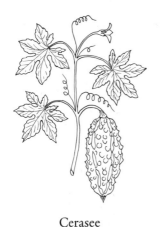

Cerasee

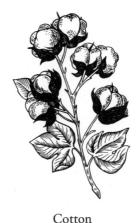

Cotton

pads with the tea, and place them over my eyes for instant relief after a long day of looking at screens.

### Guava (*Psidium guajava*)

Guava leaf is useful as a traditional medicine and as a fiber-dyeing agent. This is because of the presence of tannins. Tannins are plant compounds that impart a bitter and astringent taste, as in coffee or dry red wine. Guava leaves are used to heal diarrhea because the astringency helps tone the smooth muscles in the stomach and intestines and reduce diarrhea symptoms.

### Jigger Bush (*Tournefortia hirsutissima*)

This plant is in the same family (Boraginaceae) as borage and comfrey, and allantoin has been found in it. In the Caribbean, it is sometimes called blister bush, as it is good for getting rid of blisters, boils, and other skin conditions. A tea made from the leaves is considered very cooling. A friend named Ms. Annette said it is a good tea for people who drink a lot of alcohol, to cool their system and balance the effects of alcohol. You can put fresh leaves in room temperature water, crush them a little with your hands, and then let it infuse throughout the day for a refreshing, cooling drink.

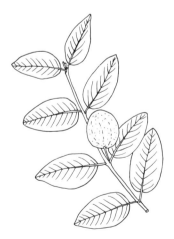

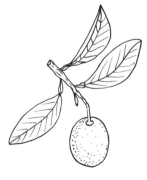

Guava (*Psidium guajava*)  Lime

## Lime (*Citrus aurantifolia*)

Limes, specifically their juice, are used for fighting colds and infections because of their vitamin C. They are also thought to clear sickness and negative energy from the air. People place cut limes in the corners of a room when someone (especially a child) cannot sleep or is not feeling well. Lime is also used to cut the taste of harsh medicines such as shark-liver oil. A woman selling shark-liver oil on a roadside in Guayaguayare, Trinidad, gave me this recipe: 1 part lime juice to 1 part shark-liver oil to 1 part honey. This is to be taken for respiratory illnesses and asthma attacks.

## Mat Root (*Aristolochia rugosa*)

This is a classic Trinidadian remedy for snakebites and scorpion stings. It is very bitter and is used in veterinary medicine as well. My friend Giselle R. said that her dog was attacked by a hive of bees and stung all over her body. She was gasping for breath and barely moving. Giselle's husband steeped a piece of mat root in hot water and gave the dog a syringeful, and the next day she was back in the bush!

## Monkey Bone or Firebush (*Hamelia patens*)

This plant is used in the treatment of menstrual issues. In the Mayan language it was known as ix-canaan, "guardian of the forest" or "healer of the forest." This name denotes its importance to Indigenous peoples.

## Obi Seed or Kola Nut (*Cola nitida*)

This is a small tree from the African continent that is used extensively in Yoruba traditional medicine and divination. The seed is chewed or brewed into a tea that gives energy and focus. A friend, Kelvin Nahkid, once brought us some obi seeds, and they were bright orange inside once they were dried. Chewing a piece the size of a pinky nail for a few minutes at a time has helped me get through the writing of this book! It gives a burst of clean energy and inspiration that lasts for hours.

## Planteh or Plantain (*Plantago major*)

Plantain, which is known as planteh in Trinidad, is a common weed from Europe to the Americas. It grew everywhere in Maryland where I grew up, and I knew of its properties as a poultice for first aid and its benefits as a tea. However, in Trinidad, my Great-Aunt Doris pointed out that it is known for washing the eyes and helping with cataracts, glaucoma, and other kinds of eye inflammation. A tea is made from the leaves, and you are supposed to drink it and use it as an eyewash for at least a week to see improvement.

## Pussley or Purslane (*Portulaca oleracea*)

This is a common roadside and farmscape weed. It is a very nutritious addition to salads, chutneys, and soups.

## Roucou (*Bixa orellana*)

Roucou is also known as achiote and annatto in different regions. Most people know it as a food coloring and additive. Others know it as a body and fiber dye. Not as many know that it has medicinal benefits.

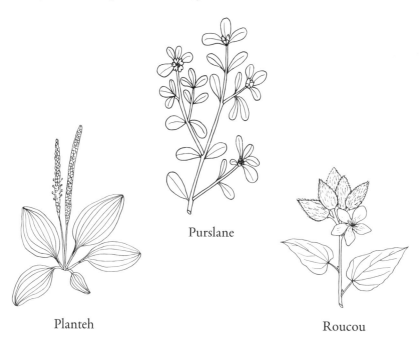

Purslane

Planteh

Roucou

The red seeds can be boiled into a tea that helps treat fevers (especially in malaria and dengue). According to ethnobotanist Francis Morean, a decoction of the root is used in the treatment of diabetes. My favorite way to use it is by infusing it into castor oil or coconut oil and using as a lip tint.

### Seed Under Leaf (*Chanca piedra*)

This plant is also called stone breaker because it works well on kidney stones and flushing out the kidneys. A woman once told me that her father mentioned it should not be drunk for long periods of time because it can have adverse effects, so she said to use it with caution.

### Soapvine (*Gouania* spp.)

This plant contains a lot of saponins and can be used to make soap when needed. This is done by rubbing the leaves together and crushing them underwater until they suds up. The smaller twigs on the vine can be broken off and used as excellent chewsticks, which have a minty flavor. The chewstick sudses up in your mouth very quickly. Jamaicans are known for powdering it and using the powder as toothpaste.

### Wild Senna (*Cassia alata*)

Wild senna is used as a tea or a bath for skin issues. It is especially effective for fungal skin issues, according to "A Catalogue of the Medicinal Plants of the Arima Valley, Trinidad" by Francis Morean. I infuse it into a salve that I make for a friend who has lotah, a type of psoriasis. In the salve I also put caraili bush, St. John's bush, and zebapique.

## CHAPTER 4

# BUSH TEAS, BUSH BATHS, AND OTHER REMEDIES

## HARVESTING MEDICINE

Harvesting medicine is a sacred and intuitive art and skill. It takes love and intention and mindfulness. My grandmother and my mother-in-law have shared with me many stories of people with a bad mind or ill intentions picking from their plants and causing the plant to die shortly after. In the Caribbean, there is also an unspoken rule about harvesting plants after sundown. It is strictly frowned upon, unless you talk nicely to the plant and make offerings to atone for waking it up at night! Most important, give thanks and never take more than you need. Another unspoken rule is to work with and learn from a knowledgeable forager or botanist before trying to identify and harvest plants that you are not 100 percent sure about. There are many poisonous look-alikes in nature!

Timing, location, moon phase, and maturity are all relatively important for determining when to harvest plants for the highest quality and medicinal value. Of course, you can harvest something whenever you want or need to, but it will have varying degrees of efficacy. There is ancestral wisdom and science in harvesting and preserving things in their due time for maximum potency. Because botany is not one-size-fits-all, along with general guidelines it takes years of place-based experience to determine the best time to harvest.

Now I will give some *very* general rules for when to harvest different parts of the plant.

## There Is a Season for Everything

❀ **Flowers.** Pick flowers in the morning after the dew has dried. Harvest them when they are fully developed in their life cycle.

❀ **Leaves.** Harvest the leafy parts of plants before the flowers form. If you wait until a plant has flowered, the energy and nutrients will have moved into the flowers. There are plenty of plants for which you might want to harvest the leaves and flowers at the same time. Also remember that most plants like to be picked (pruned), and that can encourage new growth.

❀ **Roots.** Harvest medicinal roots after the top of the plant begins to go dormant. In northern climates, this is the fall, and in tropical climates, this would be the dry season for most plants, *but not all!*

❀ **Seeds.** Seeds need to be harvested when they are completely mature and dry, usually after the plant has fully dried down.

❀ **Barks.** Barks are best harvested at the beginning of a tree's vegetative cycle, like in the spring or the beginning of the rainy season, before the saps start flowing.

❀ **Resins.** Resins are best harvested right before or after a tree is going into a hibernation, losing leaves, or heading into winter.

BUSH TEAS, BUSH BATHS, AND OTHER REMEDIES

*"Bush medicine is a 'place-based medicine,' meaning that the medicine is based on a healthy, ongoing, balanced, ecological relationship between bush medicine practitioners and the land where they harvest and use the plant.... It requires stable, healthy ecosystems, and habitat not fragmented by development, and rising seas. When this is no longer possible, documentation becomes essential and urgent. The time for documentation is now."*[41]

## Location, Location, Location

The same species of plant grown in a virgin forest versus one grown in a marginal wasteland will have different minerals and micronutrients.

- **Hills versus flats.** If I have a choice of whether to harvest the same plant on a hill or a flat, I like to harvest on the hill. And although this is purely anecdotal, I believe that herbs in the Northern Range of Trinidad hit differently from the same herbs in other areas.

- **Be careful of wastewater.** Do not harvest directly from the side of houses or roads or in drains that lead from houses or carry wastewater.

- **Avoid chemicals.** Do not harvest in areas that are sprayed with chemicals. Even though parks often have wonderful wild weeds, it behooves you to know the park maintenance practices.

- **Location of the sun.** Harvest barks from the east side of trees, which receive the morning sun, to help the tree heal itself faster.

---

41  Jeffrey Holt McCormack et al., *Bush Medicine of the Bahamas: A Cross-Cultural Perspective from San Salvador Island, Including Pharmacology and Oral Histories* (JHM Designs, 2011).

# Harvesting by the Moon

Plants' energies flow with lunar phases, traveling upward during the waxing moon and downward during the waning moon. Think of how the tides pull water, and it will help you visualize how that affects plants, which are full of water.

✿ **Full moon.** When the moon is full, it draws energy to the uppermost part of the plant. Flowers, leaves, and seeds should be harvested during the waxing or full moon.

✿ **New moon.** When it's a new moon, the energy is found deep within the roots and seeds. Roots and rhizomes are more potent during the waning or new moon.

I love studying biodynamics, and I recommend getting the *Stella Natura Biodynamic Planting Calendar* (available online) to find out good times to harvest and do different garden activities based on lunar and planetary cycles.

Again, all of this is a rough guide. It takes experience, research, and observation of your environment and plant cycles to truly learn the best time to harvest.

# Making Medicine

Medicine making is much like cooking. There are no exact recipes, and every chef imparts their own flavor and magic to the remedy or recipe. In Caribbean households and families, where the oral tradition is strong but the written record is sparse, we are left with very few exact remedies. After interviewing many elders, I have learned to stop asking them about quantities of herbs, the time to be spent steeping or soaking herbs, or how often to take a medicine and for how long. I am often met with "Feel it out," "Take a little, then go from there," or "Steep until it has a nice color." I enjoy hearing what isn't said. They are telling us to use our senses—our common sense and our intuition.

BUSH TEAS, BUSH BATHS, AND OTHER REMEDIES

Caribbean herbalism leans a lot on ritual, superstition, prayer, and intuition. For example, when you are lucky enough to learn the specific number of leaves needed in a cup of hot water, it will often be an odd number, like three, five, or seven. Also, if you ask about the regimen for a treatment, a common answer might be to take it three times a day for five days. Odd numbers have been considered lucky or divine from time immemorial, and they have been brought into Caribbean herbalism from different cultures.

> You get up in the morning and you hoarse. Get a ripe, a green, a half ripe leaf of patchouli. Draw it or boil it. Strain and drink a teacup 3 times a day. My grandmother used to say when you making tea for cold, you break according to the length. A short piece of branch what you draw, now you drink.
>
> If you want—according to the strength—you add an extra leaf lunchtime and a fifth leaf in the evening. After the first day that you drink that you feeling better. I used that already. If the leaves are small, break a bud of sweet cherry leaves. About two inches long and add to the patchouli. It has no taste, even if you add the sweet cherry leaves to leaves of patchouli is no harm. Grandmother says to use odd numbers of leaves or branches 3, 5, 7, or 9 or it is good to use green, half ripe and ripe leaves.

In this remedy, described by Miss Valeria Salazar and transcribed by Francis Morean, she tells you to drink a cup of tea three times a day and says that her grandmother taught her to use odd numbers of leaves or branches. She describes how to make a tea last throughout the day by adding leaves each time you reheat it. I appreciate that she says to use the length of a branch proportionate to the length of your cold. This type of science may not be easily quantified or studied, but it is based on hundreds of years of trial and error. It may not be written, but it is passed down in our mitochondrial DNA and through our ancestors' stories.

On the following pages, I will share more about traditional Caribbean knowledge as it pertains to making bush medicine. "Bush medicine" is a wide term for all the different remedies derived from plants. It includes teas, baths, steams, syrups, alcohols, oils, and other tonics. The type of remedy you use will be based on the herb, your ailment, and how readily available the plant is. A tea isn't going to help heal the scrape on your knee, just as a topical oil will not help heal your cold.

# BUSH TEAS

People often ask me what bush tea is, as if it were a singular thing. However, it encompasses any "bush" or plant or herb that you harvest from your vicinity and steep in hot water. In the Caribbean, bush tea is usually made with fresh herbs, although some people may use dried herbs if the fresh version is not readily available. The amount of plant material collected is usually a handful for a pot of water when dealing with gentle herbs such as lemongrass or tulsi. However, with strong, pungent, or bitter herbs, the suggested dose may just be a few leaves. Often, the stronger herbs, such as zebapique (*Neurolaena lobata*), have higher concentrations of alkaloids and other compounds that have healing properties, but they can also have adverse side effects. So they must be used with caution and not for long periods of time.

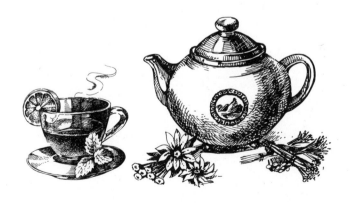

BUSH TEAS, BUSH BATHS, AND OTHER REMEDIES

Bush tea is a rite of passage in the Caribbean. Everyone has had at least one cup, given lovingly by their grandparents, a neighbor, an aunty, or a bush doctor. My daughter loves the ritual of her nightly cup of bush tea, sweetened with a little honey and diluted with fresh coconut milk. She will go outside and proudly pick the herbs she wants, which may be lemongrass (*Cymbopogon citratus*), Spanish thyme (*Plectranthus amboinicus*), or tulsi (*Ocimum* spp.). Unbeknownst to her, I may throw in a small amount of soursop (*Annona muricata*) or bois canot (*Cecropia peltata*) leaf to help her sleep even more soundly.

Teas, also known as decoctions, are one of the most common ways that herbal remedies are ingested in the Caribbean. It is common for people to drink bush tea daily in the morning or afternoon, even when they are healthy. Preventive maintenance of health and wellness is a key aspect of Caribbean herbalism, and one of the ways people upkeep their health is through bush teas. Some herbs are considered generally safe for everyday use, and it is common to grab a pinch of plants like tulsi, Spanish thyme, or lemongrass in the morning for tea. One reason herbal teas are so popular in the Caribbean is that fresh herbs are readily available year-round, and the abundant sun acts as a powerful dehydrator to dry the herbs. Teas are always made with fresh or dried plant parts that can include any of the following: leaves, stems, roots, flowers, or fruits.

A tea is a made by adding plant parts to hot water. Some herbs can be boiled, but aromatic herbs with volatile oils are best when they are steeped instead of boiled. A decoction is a very strong herbal tea that can be simmered for hours to concentrate the medicinal constituents. Both options are employed by people in the Caribbean. A stronger decoction may be stored in the refrigerator to drink over the course of a few days. A decoction also may be more likely to have more than one herb in it. A common example of a decoction is the delicious sorrel drink that in my family is simmered for up to an hour and then left overnight to steep some more.

# A Ritual for Building a Relationship with Bush Tea

One ritual that allows me to practice this type of reflection and study is my morning cup of tea. I recommend drinking the same tea for at least five days to take note of its effects on your body and to really get to know a plant medicine. Here are my steps:

1. Go for a walk in nature and notice which plants and colors and textures you are drawn to. If you can't go for a walk, think about plants or themes that keep coming up in your conversations or dreams or research.

2. Don't just see the plants; *notice* them. What is grabbing your attention? How does it make you feel to see a wild daisy or a hundred-year-old mango tree? Are you drawn to strength, calmness, color, beauty?

3. Research colors to see which of your chakras, or energy centers, are calling for attention; research the plants that you notice, to learn what they are good for. I have found that when a plant shows up in my life in a way that makes me take notice, it is usually exactly what I need, or what a loved one needs, in that moment.

4. Journal about it!

5. Either harvest the plant in an ethical fashion or order it online from a trusted source.

6. Now for the fun part—feel the plant, smell the plant, taste it in your mouth. Remark on the textures, smells, and how your body and mind react to it.

7. Using intuition or guidelines from research, decide how strong the tea will be and how much herb you will use in proportion to the hot water. Let it steep sufficiently. Let it sit all day for a decoction, or make a large pot so that you can sip throughout the day.

BUSH TEAS, BUSH BATHS, AND OTHER REMEDIES

**8.** Make your morning tea a ritual. Use your favorite mug and sit in your favorite chair. Release all deadlines and responsibilities, as your only responsibility right now is getting some good healing in the form of hot tea for ten to fifteen minutes.

**9.** Now just observe how the tea feels going down. Savor the color, texture, and smell; try to find which aromas you can detect. Take note of your breathing and the thoughts that come to you while you are drinking. For the first day or two, try not to add any ingredient like milk or sugar so that you can really get to know the plant medicine.

**10.** Repeat for five days and take note of changes in mood, skin, digestion, focus, energy. Journal about it!

**11.** Start over with a new herb or use the same herb for a longer period if you are called to. After a few months, you will have successfully added many herbs to your medicine cabinet, and you will have learned how to incorporate them into your life for your health and well-being.

# BUSH BATHS

"You need a bush bath" is a common phrase heard when someone is having a hard or transitional time in life, whether it is physical, emotional, or spiritual. I was told I needed a bush bath when ugly boils kept popping up on my skin after I got bug bites. On the other hand, my uncle was given a bush bath when he was down on his luck and getting in trouble with the law. In Trinidad, when talking politics, I have often heard "This country needs a bush bath!"

A bush bath is another commonplace ritual or activity in the Caribbean. Just as with bush tea, a bush bath can be made with a variety of herbs, depending on the ailment. The skin is the largest organ of the body and has immense absorptive ability, so our ancestors were wise to use the skin as an access point for the ingestion of herbs. Humans have been bathing with tea for just as long as they have been drinking it! Herbs are infused in a bathtub or bucket and used to treat anything from eczema to sore muscles to maljo (evil eye). Bush baths are especially indicated for babies and children, who may not be as prone to ingest these herbal medicines orally but who will happily bathe in those same herbs.

A bush bath can be performed on oneself, but in the past it was most likely done by an elder with experience, an herbal practitioner, or an Obeah person. Many Caribbeans have loving memories of their grandmother or mother soaking them in various herbs and using the actual herbs to scrub their skin while in the bath or taking a bundle of herbs and "beating" them on their body. The person receiving the bath may be seated in a tub infused with herbs or standing as the herbal infusion is poured onto their head and body. This can be done for a physical or spiritual ailment. In the case of a spiritual ailment, the person leading the ceremony will sing or recite prayers, and depending on their spiritual tradition, they may call on spirits.

The herbs may be infused into water by making a strong decoction and adding it to bathwater. Another way the plants may release their healing properties into the water is by being crushed and massaged in the water. I enjoy this type of bush bath the most because you get to infuse your energy, prayers, and intentions into the bath. When you use the crushing method, the "bath" water should be left to soak up the sun's energy to heat it and further infuse the herbs for a few hours before using. Also, for some people, the herbs may be left in the water, and for others, they may be strained out. Here are three bush bath scenarios to give you an idea of how they are performed.

1. A large pot of water will simmer on the stove with a few handfuls of different herbs. This can be made much stronger than a tea for drinking because it will be diluted. This infusion can be poured into a bathtub, and the "patient" can soak in the water for as long as needed. In Western society, this may remind people of an Epsom salt bath or a bath infused with lavender for its calming effects.

BUSH TEAS, BUSH BATHS, AND OTHER REMEDIES 109

2. Instead of the infusion of herbs being poured into a bathtub, the patient may be standing or sitting in a chair while the infusion is poured all over their body. In this instance, it is likely that the person may also use handfuls of the plant material to scrub their body, or a practitioner may rub and pound the herbs over the person's body and especially on afflicted areas.

3. A bush bath may also be done by a river or a body of water. In this case, the practitioner would harvest large bundles of herbs that can easily be held in the hand. The herbs will be splashed in the water and then rubbed and pounded on the person's skin. River and ocean water is thought to have its own healing properties, especially in the spiritual sense of washing away bad spirits or ill fortune.

My uncle once told me about his experience of receiving a bush bath from a family member. He had succumbed to drug addiction for most of his adult life, and he was always trying to get on the right footing, but he was also constantly slipping. He was in and out of group homes, and his health was failing as a result of years of chronic drug use. In our family, it was always thought that his afflictions had a psychospiritual nature because of trauma he experienced during his formative childhood years. Generally, nothing worked to keep him on the straight path, but everyone loved him dearly and prayed for him incessantly because he was truly a good person who would help anyone in need.

For his bush bath, he was stripped down to his underwear, and the elder woman had a bucket of water with plants submerged in it. The herbs he remembered were black sage (*Cordia curassavica*), gully root or guinea hen weed (*Petiveria alliacea*), sweet broom (*Scoparia dulcis*), lime, rosemary (*Salvia rosmarinus*), and blue soap. He was beaten on the back, chest, arms, legs, and temples with wads of plant material, and she also used a cocoyea broom, made with the dried and stripped leaves of a coconut tree (*Cocos nucifera*) to whack him all over his body. The variety of physical sensations helped to seal the prayers and hymns that were spoken over him. He claims, and the family noticed, that the bath worked! He was on the straight and narrow for a long while after his bush bath, and in conversations you could see and feel the shift in his spirit.

On the other hand, for a physical ailment like eczema, the herbs used will be things like cerasee (*Momordica charantia*) or wild senna leaves (*Cassia alata*). These herbs, when taken internally, are well known for their blood-building, anti-inflammatory, and antimicrobial properties. They help soothe and clear the symptoms of eczema. When the bush bath is for a physical ailment, it is common practice to also drink a course of the same herbs used in the bath for a few days after. Then a purge is administered, which can be as gentle as a tablespoon of aloe in the morning and evening for three days or something stronger, like drinking castor oil (*Ricinus communis*).

I utilize bush baths in my family for fevers and skin problems. Whenever my daughter has a fever, I boil a strong decoction of monkey bone or firebush (*Hamelia patens*) and sweet broom (*Scoparia dulcis*). Then I let it cool before pouring it over her. It has worked very well in the past to ease her symptoms but still let the fever do its job of fighting illness. I will also soak a towel in the mixture and lay it across her forehead, back, or chest. When we have skin issues like bug bites and rashes, I crush cooling herbs like cerasee, bois canot (*Cecropia peltata*), and jigger bush (*Tournefortia hirsutissima*). I then gently rub them on our skin and pour the water over our bodies. I do this as the last step of bathing, and then we air-dry to allow maximum absorption.

# ROOT TONICS

> *"[It depends on the] amount of different things you put in it, for a tea [you] just [put a plant like] sarsaparilla, ramoon, chainey root. For a tonic you put more things, 20 different something, bark and roots."*[42]

A root tonic is a metaphor for Caribbean culture. The variety of inputs, the strong flavor, the healing are all inherently Caribbean. And it has roots in all the cultures that inhabit these beautiful islands. A bottle may contain dozens of herbs. Herbs that may have originated in the Americas, like guinea hen weed; or in Europe, like comfrey; or in Africa, like obi seed, will all inhabit the same bottle and mix and meld in synergistic ways.

> *"The Maroons ran away and survived in the forests and they started the tradition [of boiling root tonics]. But their knowledge originated out of Africa. They tapped into the knowledge in order to survive."*[43]

Root tonics have deep roots in Jamaican and Rasta culture but are also found in different forms throughout the Caribbean. Some basic components are (1) a wide variety of synergistic herbs in the form of roots, barks, leaves, and seeds; (2) a curing or fermenting process; (3) the addition of wine, rum, sugar, honey, or molasses; and (4) a long boiling period, preferably in a large pot in an outdoor fire.

The long boiling period is necessary because roots and barks take more time and heat to release their healing properties. Another practice to maximize extraction of constituents is to soak the roots and barks in

---

42   I. Vandebroek et al., "Root Tonics and Resilience: Building Strength, Health, and Heritage in Jamaica," *Frontiers in Sustainable Food Systems* 5 (February 22, 2021), doi: 10.3389/fsufs.2021.640171.
43   Vandebroek et al., "Root Tonics and Resilience."

water overnight or for a day to soften the plant cell walls. A tonic will generally not have delicate or highly aromatic (high volatile oil) plants like mint. Those are better steeped instead of boiled.

Tonics may or may not include a fermentation process. This is done by adding ingredients like ginger or raisins to kick-start fermentation and leaving the bottle to age for days or weeks. This is important if you want a shelf-stable product. You can also achieve shelf stability by adding alcohol to your tonic.

# WINES

My first time being gifted a bottle of homemade herbal wine was from an elder woman named Mrs. Horsford in Parlatuvier, Tobago. I was accompanying ethnobotanist Francis Morean while he was doing field research on hill rice by interviewing elders. When talking about farming and hill rice, herbal use inevitably comes up. As we walked into her yard, I saw a healthy green plant with what looked like small warts on it. I asked her what it was. She said it was named cure-for-all, and Francis gave me its other common name, geritout (*Pluchea carolinensis*). She remarked that people came from all over to buy it for asthma, coughs, colds, and other infections.

This was my introduction to herbal wines, and it fascinated me. It made so much sense to harness and preserve the healing power of an herb through fermentation, which yields its own benefits. In Trinidad and Tobago, almost any plant or fruit is turned into wine by skillful hands. I have tasted ganja (*Cannabis indica*) wine, hog plum wine, sorrel wine, pineapple wine, mango wine, star fruit wine, elderflower wine, jamoon wine. You get the point!

These wines are generally made from the herb or flower with sugar, the juice of a fruit, a strong infusion of the plant material, and yeast. Often, ginger or raisins may be put in for their medicinal benefits and their ability to aid in the fermentation. Boiling water is poured over the herbs, and they are left to steep overnight. The herbs are strained out, then the sugar, fruits, yeast, and ginger or raisins are added and left to ferment. In seven to twenty-one days, you have wine. Most herbal and fruit wine makers leave their wines to age for months or years, and they judge each other's wines by how see-through the resulting liquid is and the alcohol content.

# TINCTURES

My first introduction to making herbal medicine for others was in the form of tinctures. I regularly made teas for myself and had begun experimenting with soaking our fall harvests in Everclear alcohol. One year, after planting oats as a cover crop on my farm on the Eastern Shore of Maryland, I noticed that the oats were in a milky phase (the phase between vegetative and seed formation). I had a few herbalist friends who recommended it for nervous system restoration and overall vitality. Since the oats were a cover crop and we did not want them to go to seed, it made perfect sense for me to harvest the milky oat tops before they hardened and turned to a seed that could become an unwanted weed.

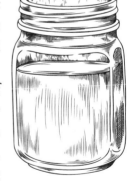

I went to the store, bought a big bottle of Everclear, and filled a large mason jar halfway full of fresh milky oats. Then I poured the alcohol on top, and my first tincture was started. I tinctured it on a new moon, and I strained it on a full moon two months later. I bottled it, gave it away to friends, and used it myself to restore my nervous system after a stressful season and heartache. I was hooked on this new way to preserve plants and ingest medicine, and it has become one of my favorite ways to share herbal medicine.

The best alcohol to use for tinctures is 190 proof. This allows you to dilute it to the percentage of alcohol you desire in the final product. For example, if you are using fresh herbs, the alcohol must be at least 80 proof, or you risk the tincture not being properly preserved. You can dilute a 190 proof alcohol to 80 proof by diluting with distilled or spring water. If you are using fresh herbs that still have moisture, you should use the highest-proof alcohol you can find. This is because the water content in the herbs will dilute the alcohol content of the finished product. Use alcohol without additives because additives decrease the alcohol's extracting ability.

Now that I live in Trinidad, my method remains the same, but the plants differ. I use soursop leaf tincture as a nervine instead of milky oats. I draw on the medicinal benefits of bitter plants by using papaya leaf instead of dandelion root. The Caribbean does not have a culture of making tinctures in the sense of a single herb soaked in alcohol and strained. Instead, there is a culture of tonics that may be a combination of roots, barks, and leaves soaked in overproof rum indefinitely. As opposed to straining out the plant material, Caribbean tonics may be soaked for years and sometimes decades. Alcohol and fresh herbs are added over time to replenish the bottle.

In many Caribbean countries, a bush rum is traditionally distilled using molasses, which itself is thought to have healing benefits. Rum is a preferred alcohol for some traditional herbal practitioners. Some alcohols that may be used are puncheon rum, White Oak, Wray & Nephew, or any common rum in a particular country. Alcohol works by extracting the active ingredients of a plant into a solvent (a substance that easily dissolves things). The longer it sits, the more potent it becomes. It also helps to cut up or blend the plant materials in advance so there is more surface area for the alcohol to extract the medicinal properties. Generally, roots, stems, and barks will need to be soaked longer than leaves.

BUSH TEAS, BUSH BATHS, AND OTHER REMEDIES

One alcohol infusion that I use often is babash (bush rum) with tobacco leaves, rosemary leaves, ginger root, camphor, and coconut oil. A man named Hulk in South Trinidad told me that he uses this combination whenever he has a head cold, to get rid of any and all congestion. He told me to put some on my crown and temples before bed and then cover my head. He recommended doing this for three nights in a row and then to purge by drinking a little castor oil for three days to get rid of any cold in the body. I use this now for headaches or fever, and I also learned that rubbing it on my throat and chest helps alleviate cough or respiratory symptoms at night. It works almost instantly when I massage it gently on my sinus pathways along my temples and under my eyes.

As you can see, alcohol is a versatile way to preserve and ingest herbal medicine. To ingest a tincture, the dosage is generally one to three dropperfuls per day. For a tonic, the dosage is generally half to a full shot glass per day. You can add alcohol-based herbal medicines to your tea, water, or juice to make them more palatable.

## How to Make a Simple Tincture

This is considered a folk method for making a tincture. There are more standardized ways of creating tinctures using specific ratios of plant matter, alcohol, and water to create a desired potency.

**1.** If you are using fresh herbs, chop them finely. If you are using dried herbs, grind them to a coarse powder. You can also use a mortar and pestle.

**2.** Put the herbs in a glass jar and make sure to label it with the date and the type of herbs.

**3.** Add enough alcohol to cover the herbs.

**4.** Add the cover or lid and put the jar in a dark area at room temperature.

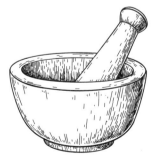

**5.** Shake daily, or whenever you remember, to speed up the process and make a more potent extraction.

**6.** After a minimum of four weeks, strain out the herbs. You can leave the herbs in the alcohol for as long as you like.

**7.** Ideally, store the tincture in amber glass bottles away from direct sunlight.

# OILS

Oil is another substance that acts as a solvent for the medicinal compounds in plants. Essential oils, also known as volatile oils, that are present in plants such as rosemary and tree resins are generally soluble in oils such as coconut oil, cocoa butter, olive oil, and jojoba oil. Compounds such as the alkaloids in the nightshade family or mucilage in the mallow family are more soluble in water or alcohol. Therefore, you choose the medium for making your medicine depending on which properties you want to extract from a plant.

In the Caribbean, coconut oil is one of the most-used oils for medicinal purposes. The history of how coconut has traveled around the world reflects the movements of people since ancient times. Coconut is a staple of almost all tropical cultures, and it is believed to have originated in the Pacific Ocean basin as well as in the Indian Ocean basin. Scientists believe that coconuts from Polynesia were brought to the shores of Southeast Asia, East Africa, and Madagascar by Austronesian traders thousands of years ago. Coconuts were introduced into Europe by Arab traders and then into the Caribbean during the transatlantic slave trade.[44]

---

44 Diana Lutz, "Deep History of Coconuts Decoded," Washington University, Newsroom, June 24, 2011, https://source.washu.edu/2011/06/deep-history-of -coconuts-decoded.

BUSH TEAS, BUSH BATHS, AND OTHER REMEDIES

You can see why, in a Caribbean culture with deep influences from Southeast Asia, the coconut would be widely used. I learned to make coconut oil from my husband, who learned from his mother, who learned from her parents, who were descendants of Indian indentured servants who came to Trinidad in the late 1800s. Extracting the oil from a dried coconut is a labor-intensive process that yields liquid gold.

Alone or infused with herbs, coconut oil is a medicinal powerhouse that treats a range of internal and external conditions. I fondly remember when my daughter was a small baby and elders inevitably advised me to rub coconut oil on the soft spot on her head and told me of the virtues of massaging her regularly with coconut oil. We used to call her coconut oil baby because she always had that aroma.

Other oils that are important in Caribbean herbalism are as follows:

❀ Castor oil (*Ricinus communis*)
❀ Carapa oil (*Carapa guianensis*)
❀ Palm oil
❀ Cocoa butter (*Theobroma cacao*)
❀ Sesame oil
❀ Mustard oil

The type of oil is just as important as the herbs you plan to infuse into it. Herb-infused oils can be ingested in small doses or applied topically for rashes, muscle pain, wound care, headaches, eczema, or bug bites. Herbs that may be used to target muscle pain or arthritis are cayenne, turmeric, clove, bay leaf, and nutmeg. Herbs that may be in a skin cream would be neem, turmeric, papaya, cerasee, or comfrey. When making an herbal oil for oil pulling (a method of cleansing the mouth, gums, and teeth), herbs such as clove, cayenne, rosemary, or mint may be used.

There are two general methods for infusing an herb into an oil. They both start with dried herbs. Properly dried herbs make a more shelf-stable product, since moisture promotes the growth of bacteria. Properly stored oils can last for years, and often the herbs will have their own antimicrobial properties that help preserve the oil. The herbs should be crushed, blended, or pounded to break them up into smaller pieces. Here is where the two methods differ. One uses a stovetop to heat and speed up the infusion. The other uses time and sometimes solar energy to slowly infuse the herbs.

With the abundance of solar energy in the Caribbean, it is the most common method of extracting herbs into oils. The heat from the sun helps catalyze the process. It is also believed that light and heat from the sun can extract and imbue properties that would not be there with heat alone. You will need a glass jar, which you will fill about three-quarters full with plant material. Then add your oil of choice to cover the herbs, leaving at least one inch of space between the liquid and the lid to allow for expansion. Close the lid and place the jar in a spot that receives adequate sunlight daily. You can bring it inside at night if needed. Allow at least two weeks for the infusion, and then strain it through cheesecloth. Often, I strain only what is needed and leave the herbs soaking in the oil for months at a time to make a stronger oil. Be careful to always make sure the herbs are fully submerged in the oil to prevent spoilage.

If you are using applied heat, prepare a double boiler system or set a Crockpot to low heat. Place the herbs in the oil and heat the mixture for one to eight hours, depending on the desired strength. Once the oil cools down, strain it through cheesecloth and store the oil in a glass container. A heavy sludge may settle at the bottom; the next day, you can pour off the oil on top for a cleaner finished product. For both methods, a ratio of 1 part herbs to 5 parts oil is sufficient for a potent herb. For example, to make a turmeric-infused oil, use 100 grams of turmeric to 500 milliliters of oil.

The following are some of the common ways herbal oils are used:

❀ They can be applied directly to a bug bite, rash, ache, or pain.

❀ They can be heated and massaged into an affected area.

- They can be slathered on an affected area, followed by application of a warm compress, such as a warm water bottle or a warm piece of flannel.

- To make a salve, the herbal oil can be mixed with something with a higher melting point, such as beeswax or cocoa butter. A general recipe for a good salve is two parts liquid oil to one part beeswax or cocoa butter. You can combine all oils, waxes, or butters in a double boiler to melt them and then carefully pour them into a jar. Adjust the ratios to get the consistency you want.

- To make a cream, you will need about one cup of distilled water or herbal tea at room temperature, one cup of infused oil, and one ounce of melted beeswax. Melt the beeswax into the oil in a double boiler. When the mixture has cooled for three to five minutes, you can begin slowly adding the water or tea to the oil and beeswax while whisking with a fork or using a handheld blender. Keep mixing until your mixture has a creamy consistency, and stop adding water when you get to that point.

## CHAPTER 5

# INTERVIEWS AND BOTANICAL MUSINGS

## EXPERIENCES OF A MIDWIFE AND HILL RICE FARMER: ALICE PRENTIS

The following is an excerpt from an interview conducted by Aleya Fraser and Francis Morean, transcribed by Francis Morean.

I have been living on this spot for more than forty years. The Lord brought me here. I wanted to pull out from here and go back to Clarke-Rochard Road, but the Lord told me to stay here. My parents' home was in Clarke-Rochard Road.

Before here I was living in a little galvanize shed in the forest in Santoo Trace in Buenos Ayres.

I was around fifty years old at the time and I stayed there for four years. I came here when I had fifty-five years. In there I planted pumpkins, pigeon peas, cassava, yam. I did not plant any rice. I and sweet potato don't agree.

I lost my good rice seeds. Since years ago I could not plant the good rice seeds that I had at the time. I gave it to my son but he did not plant it. My husband was sick so I could not go in the garden. The doctor had told me not to leave him unattended. That rice was a broad, fat grain and it tasted better. The variety I have now was sent to me by a fellow from Moruga. But it is not the one I had been looking for.

My mother was Theodora Lewis. She was born up St. Mary's. She was a midwife. When I had twelve years I began going out with her. One time she went somewhere quite down in the back of Penal. Sometimes when she is rubbing the woman I am there with her. I was the last, the behe in the midst.

She used to ask them for a razor blade and she used to put the razor blade to boil for about five minutes, and when it boiled she used to take it out of the boiling water. Then she milked the navel string. She milked a certain part of the navel string. She milked it, milked it until it got flat. Then she tied it and then she cut it. About an inch and a half. She used to bury the afterbirth. Sometimes the girl's mother-in-law would wrap it in newspaper and then buried it.

I didn't want this walk. I did not want this work at all. I said "Who me?" I didn't want this work. Then I started to get the instinct to boil bush. First, I did not want this work that at first I used to go by my neighbor to do it. Eventually my husband began to complain.

I does rub the children with nara. I fix hasooli. I does jharay them with the coconut broom. The old people did teach me those prayers. The heavenly people. When I do not know something I does ask them.

The next thing they told me is not to charge people. Whatever they gave me was to take it. I sitting down here and I heard a voice. I was told to attend to a man who had problems. I keep me

122                                                          CARIBBEAN HERBALISM

hand right there until he stopped bawling. You know it was gas all over the man body.

The first time I put a woman to bed with a baby was with my stepmother. She was pregnant. She was living Ramsabag Trace. She was already crowning. So I called for some oil and I soaked the passageway and I called for a coconut broom and I just passed it on her and I used prayers. I cut the navel string and I told her. I was forty-eight years.

Sometimes you have five women to deal with at the same time. Sometimes you have to deal with three at the same time.

They have to keep away from black eye peas, red beans and all those things because they causes the baby to puff. No pepper. That causes a lot of heat to break out all over the child's skin. No cassava, no deer meat. That does dry up the milk. Pregnant women should not drink the vervine.

The seim (a type of legume) is good to eat during pregnancy. Soups with chicken foot, pumpkin, carrots, a lot of garlic and onions. The more soups the better. But do not use the shado beni, the cut-and-throw or what they call it, that does cause the pressure to raise.

You can boil the root of the shado beni and drink it from three days after delivery if you feeling any pain and you want to clean out the clot blood.

As a mother, the milk does start to leak or otherwise your back does start to hurt you.

Since bush rum was two dollars a bottle I used to make it.

I made in the bush in Ayres. Then when I went down to Buenos Ayres I start to make and a good bit of people used to follow me. Use ripe fig, pine, cane, anything, but I did not put of all that. I used to get two to three pitch oil tins of rum from one boil. I used to carry rum in the night, all Mayaro to sell.

One night the van shut down in Mayo right in front of a policeman and he came and helped me to fix the van. After he

INTERVIEWS AND BOTANICAL MUSINGS

fixed it I drove off. Another time I was going to Sando and they stopped me. An Inspector from the Penal Police Station used to send a car to warn me when they planning to raid me. So I used to go in Ayres and take out the gallon bottles of the rum and I placed them in the river or in the root of the immortelle. The police did not go there to search.

I used to tell the police, "All you now reach? What take all you so long?"

A few times police came banging on my door. They came one morning about eleven o'clock and told me that they were looking for bush rum.

Other women did it as well, but it was not as good as mine.

If it coming out from the cooler, it is not good. You have to pull out the wood at that stage. It had to come cool.

Some women, their boilers smoking and they done collecting the rum. But I allowed the rum to come cool. Take your time and let the rum cook good. You can be drinking the rum right here and nobody would know. It had no strong smell.

Mata burro makes a nice bush rum.

I drank bush rum right through my pregnancies with my children.

I boiled bush rum for over five to six years and send my children to college. I don't put pomeracs. I quicker put the mataburro and pine and cane.

I born and grow in hill rice because my mother used to plant hill rice. They used to plant acres of hill rice.

That was in Platanique Forest. You going towards Penal and then when you reach Clarke Road elementary school, you go straight. In there was big forest. They used to cut down as much lands as they wanted. Nobody interfered with them. But they did not cut the good trees like mora, balata, water cedar and so on.

They used to plant the Black Hen rice one side. They did not want them to mix up. But both varieties were good. The Black

Hen rice was black right through on the outside. You don't see that again. And the birds did not use to pick that one.

Long ago here had a lot of coral snakes and mapepire (types of poisonous snakes).

Sometimes when I was living in Buenos Ayres I used to hear a noise by the building. When I woke up to check, it most times was a snake. Like the Holy Spirit used to wake me in time.

The machete and the horsewhip smells fresh but the mapepire has a fainty, fainty scent.

A woman came to see me from as far as Tabaquite. She never had a child and when she was having pains her husband brought her to see me. When I checked her I realised that she was ready to deliver and I had to deliver the child one time. I cut her navel string.

I use sweet man bush to bathe the babies.

My husband used to tell me to get up and mark the date when he knew I was pregnant. But we did not know anything when we first got pregnant. I work hard too bad. I used to have to work bareback even when I had to cut down roseau. Once, when I was in Buenos Ayres, a whole roseau tree fell on my back. I had to call a man to help me to remove the branches.

I used to cut and tote barefooted a truckload and a half of big nice bunches of bananas down in Platanique.

In those days I was fat like a whip, but I could have work too bad. When my husband heard what I had been doing in there by myself, he could not believe it. I had orange, portugal, coffee, limes, fig, yams, coconut, all kinds of thing. I spent years working on that garden. I had it clean and well maintained with my cutlass. We did not know anything about spraying in those days. I have eight acres close to the cemetery. I bought that with bush rum money. I made good use of that money.

INTERVIEWS AND BOTANICAL MUSINGS

# BOTANICAL MUSINGS ON GENIPA

One of my favorite things to research is a plant's origin story. Where is it considered native, and how was this plant tied to the Indigenous people who first discovered and used it? What names did they call it, and did it have a role in their cosmology?

Within its native habitat, genipa or jagua (*Genipa americana*) was and is used to summon strength, give protection in war, induce transformation, attract mates, and connect to spirits, among other things. It is a very multifaceted and dynamic fruit, and it is an important part of rituals throughout the Amazon basin and the Caribbean, including present-day Venezuela, Peru, Mexico, Puerto Rico, Suriname, Guyana, Trinidad, Ecuador, Panama, Brazil, and Colombia.

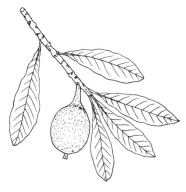

*Genipa americana*

My research allows me to have a closer relationship with plants and helps me understand their cultural and medicinal uses on another level. *Genipa americana* got its Latin nomenclature from the Portuguese European interpretation of how the Tupi language group of South Americans pronounced andï 'pawa" as yanipa.[45]

In Ecuador, it would have been a word that sounded more like wituk (now huito) and corresponded to an origin myth about two beautiful sisters, Wituk (*Genipa americana*) and Manduru (*Bixa orellana*), who transformed the various first beings into various species of plants and

---

45   A. Pamies et al., "'Fruits Are Results': On the Interaction Between Universal Archi-Metaphors, Ethno-Specific Culturemes and Phraseology," *Journal of Social Sciences* 11, no. 3 (March 2015): 227–47, doi: 10.3844/jssp.2015.227.247.

animals by painting them various shades of red, reddish brown, and black. Both genipa and roucou (*Bixa orellana*) are still used today as part of traditions dating back thousands of years in Indigenous cultures for protection (spiritually and from insects) and decoration (ritual and everyday).

My journey with genipa began when it was mentioned in a WhatsApp group where someone posted the picture and asked for an ID. It looked familiar to me, and I ended up identifying it a few times in various places. However, it was often at the overripe stage once the fruits had fallen to the ground. The tree grows very tall and straight, and most leaves and fruits are at the top. It forces you to look up!

The fruit is ripe once it is soft and pungent. The smell is unique and inviting yet wild and musky. One of its names is monkey apple because the seeds are dispersed by howler and capuchin monkeys. The ripe fruit has uses as a bronchodilator and respiratory aid, among others, and is made into juices, ice cream, fermented drinks, syrups, and liquors. For example, in Puerto Rico, it is sliced and put in a jar of water with sugar to make a drink like lemonade, and sometimes it is left for a few days to ferment. Genipa is a fruit high in vitamin B and minerals such as iron, calcium, and phosphorus and proteins, lipids, and fibers.

> *"In Peru, the huitoshado or huitochado—brandy made from sugar cane loaded with fruit pieces and flavored with honey from wild bees—is very popular. It is believed that the drink strengthens the organism, and relieves it from the inner cold. In addition, it has even been reported that it counteracts sexual dysfunction to the elderly people."*[46]

Once I felt confident identifying the tree by its fallen fruits, leaves, and bark, I was able to observe the genipa trees around me for a full year,

---

46    J. Tournon et al., "Ethnobotany of the Shipibo-Konibo," *Folia* 7, no. 6 (2014): 78–107, https://doi.mendelu.cz/artkey/doi-990002-8200_Ethnobotany-of-the-Shipibo-Konibo.php.

from watching their fragrant and velvety yellow flowers being visited by all manner of insect pollinators to seeing fruit form. The round green fruit takes months and months to mature and ripen.

It is a semi-deciduous tree, so in a particularly dry season or climate, the leaves start to yellow and fall off to conserve water. In other climates or when growing close to sources of water, it rarely loses its leaves. Interestingly enough, one of its methods of dispersal is that the unripe fruits can float, and they can remain viable while submerged in water for up to four months as well as mature away from the mother tree. They often float down streams or rivers, and when they mature, a change in density causes them to sink to the bottom. When the streambed dries up, they germinate.

Although the first trees I found were too tall for me to harvest unripe fruits from, I soon found an abundance of trees somewhere else, in Loango, Trinidad. Their fruits could be harvested by standing on a car or using a long pole with a knife attached. It is a blessing that the fruits take so long to ripen because it is in the unripe stage that they offer up their beautiful, mystic blue-black dye.

The dye is one of the most magical botanical products I have ever encountered. "To make the unseen seen" is a phrase that runs through my head when I am using the dye. This is because the juice from the unripe fruit is light gray when it is squeezed from the fruit, is clear when it goes onto your skin, and slowly reveals its dark, intoxicating color and pattern over the course of twelve hours. It is considered a permanent dye, as it permanently bonds with collagen protein in your top layer of skin and fades only as your epidermis sheds and renews itself over the course of one to two weeks. Fascinating!

Genipa is a member of the Rubiaceae family, along with coffee, ixora, and gardenia. Genipa and gardenia both contain the phytopigment genipin, which gives off its lovely color so easily to the proteins in our skin. Genipin is initially colorless, but in the presence of oxygen it reacts with amines and proteins in your epidermis to produce bluish-violet pigments. While reacting with your skin, it creates linkages in collagen molecules. For this reason, it is being researched in the fields of tissue regeneration and dentistry.

# DEALING WITH DENGUE: FROM PAPAYA TO PRAYERS

Dengue is an infectious disease spread by the bite of an infected mosquito. In some places, it used to be known as breakbone fever. This is because of the intense bone and joint pain, which makes an infected person feel as if their bones are breaking, and the intense fever, which can last for a week or more.

There were thousands of cases in Trinidad in 2024, in contrast to the fifty-seven cases reported in 2023. Apparently this is a worldwide issue, and according to the World Health Organization's website, the number of reported dengue cases has doubled each year since 2021, with over 12.3 million cases for the year already by August 2024.

Prevention and protection are the only two sure ways to avoid getting dengue. You must try to eliminate any breeding grounds for the *Aedes* species of mosquito by disposing of, upturning, or putting mosquito-proof coverings on anything that can collect water. Keeping bush and undergrowth low and cleaning drains and gutters also helps the flow of water. Mosquitoes need standing water to breed, so as long as water is flowing, it will not harbor them. These measures may seem simple, but dengue spreads in neighborhoods and environments where there are abandoned houses, cars, and yards as well as in swampy areas with poor drainage. Some people advocate for chemically spraying neighborhoods and breeding grounds, but those efforts do not show long-lasting effects. Instead, large-scale and intensive community cleanups and updated infrastructure are needed to address any areas of standing water.

INTERVIEWS AND BOTANICAL MUSINGS

Trinidad had an especially rough time with mosquitoes in 2024. Everyone lamented that the insects were attacking in droves and were more relentless than ever. This could have been a result of the intense rainy season as well as a lack of community maintenance. My grandmother's caregiver was the first person who I learned of having dengue. She was sent to the hospital, and her platelet counts dropped. It took her over three weeks to fully recover. I then started hearing about case after case, often involving hospitalization, and even a few deaths. Most people felt that the media had just stopped reporting on it and the number of cases and deaths must be much higher than official numbers.

The *Aedes* mosquitoes that carry dengue fly only a few hundred feet from their breeding grounds. This is why whole families or whole communities are affected, as a mosquito will bite an infected person and keep hopping around for its approximately two-week adult life as a bloodsucking machine. This made us feel relatively safe, as we live a few hundred feet from our nearest neighbors, so all of our mosquitoes would technically not be able to bite anyone else and bring the disease back to us. One thing we did not do was take extra precautions to avoid being bitten while out in public places or mosquito hot spots.

Unfortunately, my husband did fall ill with dengue. We had come home after an herbal workshop when he said he was exhausted and needed to go to bed early. The next morning, he told me that he had delirious dreams and woke up exhausted, with a little nausea. We thought he had a stomach bug that was going around, but he never threw up and did not have any other gastrointestinal symptoms. When his joint pains, headaches, and sudden, persistent fever kicked in, we started to feel it might be dengue. His other major symptom was complete loss of appetite.

# Herbal Regimen

The following day, I took my daughter to the library and found a reference book called *Amazing Power of Healing Plants* by Reinaldo Sosa Gómez. I opened the book, and to my surprise I landed on the page about dengue. It described my husband's symptoms to a T and offered some advice and herbs to use, so I took photographs of the pages and got to work on a healing regimen. It is important to know what classic dengue is, as opposed to hemorrhagic dengue, to assess whether the disease is worsening or getting better. For example, a high fever can persist for up to seven days, but one should worry if it lasts longer. If symptoms are not getting better by seven to ten days, the disease may be progressing and hospital treatment may be required to assess hydration, nutritional status, and blood platelet levels. If you are experiencing any abnormal bleeding from the gums or nose or blood in your feces or vomit, you need to seek professional help. Coupled with fever and joint pain, those are signs of hemorrhagic dengue, which can be fatal.

We had on hand a few of the herbs mentioned in the book for fever. One was roucou or annatto (*Bixa orellana*). The book recommended making a tea of the red seeds and drinking it. We also had lemongrass, known in Trinidad as fever grass, which was of course recommended to support the fever process. I made a strong infusion of roucou seeds, zebapique (*Neurolaena lobata*), lemongrass (*Cymbopogon citratus*), lani bois (*Piper marginatum*), Spanish thyme (*Plectranthus amboinicus*), ginger (*Zingiber officinale*), and gully root (*Petiveria alliacea*), which he drank regularly throughout the day. This concoction gave him micronutrients to help fuel his cells and also alkaloids, tannins, and flavonoids, which have anti-inflammatory, blood-building, antimicrobial, and immune system boosting actions.

Pawpaw, also known as papaya (*Carica papaya*), is medicinal from the leaves to the fruits to the seeds. For acute viral infections, it is advised to juice the leaves for the strongest medicine. You can also make tea of the leaves, which is gentler but still effective. I would not recommend taking it for more than five days in a row because it is a strong medicine that can have side effects.

Dengue tends to suppress bone marrow activity, which is what leads to low platelet counts. To support his platelet counts and bone health, we used bone broth in *everything*. He had little appetite, but he was able to sip bone broth or drink nourishing dal (split pea soup) made with bone broth. I made sure he ate broth, soup, or fruit regularly because nutrition is needed to support healing. I also used my mortar and pestle to pound up pawpaw leaves to make a juice, which he took a small shot glass of every day for a few days. To the shot I added salt and lime juice to make the bitterness more palatable. Papaya leaves are proven to raise platelet counts during mosquito-borne illnesses and contain compounds such as quercetin, which in modern times is isolated from plants and sold as an immunotherapy.

To support overall immune health and response to infection, I like to focus on activities that support the lymphatic system and herbs or substances that support white blood cell function. One of those substances is shark-liver oil. This oil contains a compound, squalene, that elicits a strong immune response and is even used in vaccine therapies to help vaccines elicit an immune response. My thought process is to always go with the most natural route, and it's interesting to find out when a natural medicine is the basis of a modern Western pharmaceutical. So he took one tablespoonful of shark oil each day, mixed with lime juice and honey.

To support his lymphatic system, which carries white blood cells, hormones, and wastes to their appropriate places in the body, I made sure he kept moving, even when it hurt. Even in bed he had to stretch, and whenever he had a burst of energy, he went outside for some fresh air and sunlight, took a walk, or did some light yardwork. I regularly monitored his temperature, blood pressure, and heart rate to make sure they were staying within an expected range and were continually moving back toward his baseline.

All of this was reinforced by prayer and intention and love, which more often than not does a lot of the healing work. It was also important to heed the warnings of illness, which are to slow down, introspect, and remove stressors. Within a week he was back to 80 percent, and by ten days he was taking me on a road trip for my birthday. He did have to take a pain medicine and fever reducer a few times over the roughest three days, but he didn't take them regularly because his symptoms were bearable thanks to the support of the other treatments.

*It should go without saying that this is not professional medical advice. I am simply sharing my experiences in hopes that others will do their own research and use what they have available to them to support healing and recovery.*

## Prevention

Our daughter and I worked on prevention by taking smaller amounts of shark oil and bush teas. We made sure to wear long sleeves and pants when we could, and we kept Michael covered up so no mosquitoes could bite him and then bite us. I am not a fan of bug sprays and mosquito coils, but desperate times call for desperate measures. On the days when he was sick, we did burn the coil at entrances to deter mosquitoes, and we used Odomos repellent cream on our bodies. We also went through the yard, cut areas that may have been breeding grounds, and turned over all of our wheelbarrows and buckets. These measures drastically reduced the number of mosquitoes that bit us and prevented the disease from passing on to me or our daughter.

I hope you enjoyed my thought process in working through illness and healing in my family. I love being able to go into my yard and use what I have to boost our systems. I learned much of what I know by talking with elders, combing through research articles, and experiencing firsthand the healing power of herbs. All of these things also help build my intuition muscles, which guide me to the correct remedies and prayers to use.

INTERVIEWS AND BOTANICAL MUSINGS                    133

# TRADITIONAL WISDOM FROM MY MUDDA-IN-LAW: GLORIA PARRIS

The following is an excerpt from an interview conducted by Aleya Fraser, transcribed by Aleya Fraser.

The prompt for this interview was to describe her favorite herbal medicines and to recount her experiences with traditional massage. I am grateful that my daughter and husband were present for this interview so that the knowledge was passed on in our family.

> Carpenter bush. Whatever ails us, fever, headache cold. My mother would brew the carpenter bush. Say like um 2 cups of water to a handful of leaves. In those days you didn't have measuring or whatever, so you take a handful of leaves, put it in the pot and then you boil it for like 2 minutes, you turn off your stove and you drink that. Sometimes you put a little sugar in it but usually its just like that. Warm, you drink it. And whatever ails you, it heals you. I know that for sure.
>
> And then we had, we make tea with bush. Like orange peel or with a few leaves. We always boil that and we make tea. We put sugar in it or you could put a little milk.
>
> Then when you had diarrhea you use the guava leaves and a piece of the guava bark. You boil it and when you boil it the color of water changes to reddish brown and you drink it. It will stop the diarrhea. You would take it like 2x for the day and 3 days for the week and by that time you are healed and feeling better.
>
> When women had period pain, you boil carilli bush. You boil about 10 leaves in about 2 cups of water and you drink half a cup in the morning and like you drink half a cup in afternoon and half a cup in the night. So next day, you boil a new batch and whatever

CARIBBEAN HERBALISM

is left you drink out. And that help to stop the pain, carilli bush. I remember that one well.

I remember them when I was younger and used them all the time. Whenever I had pain or fever or cold we use different bush. Most of the bush gone and disappeared and then we had modern medicine. In those days you would hardly go to a doctor because money was hard and each one, teach one. Like the neighbor knows you sick, so they bring a little bush tea for you. But now you see medicine becoming available and people have more money, they prefer to go to pharmacy and get something for the fever, get something for the cold, get something for period pain or diarrhea.

Like when you have a headache, you soak your head with bay rum but nowadays you have a headache, you go to pharmacy and get panadol and your headache is gone. But in those days it was not easy like that. It was easier to get the bush medicine. But now its harder to get the bush medicine because the bush them gone, they disappear. And if you have them now, big companies take them and they make tea and they cost so much money. But it's the same bush we used when we were children. And then when scientists discover, let me make some medicine and put it on the market so people get rid of all the bush and they start using what the scientist say. The scientist say use this one.

Like with coconut oil they say was bad for you because people used to grate their OWN coconut and make their OWN oil to cook and then when other oils become available and scientists made new set of oil, they said the coconut oil was bad! Now in this 20th century they say its best for you. It's a miracle cure! But in those days, they said it was not good. They bad talk it and say it not good for you. It will give you heart attack. But cholesterol is something. We never know dat word when we was small because there was nothing like that.

INTERVIEWS AND BOTANICAL MUSINGS

Because people use natural food, natural vegetables, and natural fertilizer from the chicken pen. Everybody had a cow, some people have a goat, right. And most people had common fowl in the yard and they didn't use the chickens from these farms and eggs were local eggs. We had local goat and local pigs. We had all that. There was no freezer and fridge and supermarket like now. So everybody had fresh meat on weekend. Now you have meat 2 years in the freezer and that's what we eating now.

But bush tea was a regular thing in most homes. After school close in June/July, everybody supposed to take a purge. There was a senna tree in somebody's back yard and they would bring some for your mudda for everybody to drink. Like your whole village know, school closed, time for a purge. They would bring some and you would take some what you have and that is how it goes. So all the children in the school get purged.

I didn't do it with my children because the scientists say there is no need to do that, so we believe in science. So we never do that again. And then you listen to the news or read a magazine and they talk about its not necessary, it weaken the lining of your stomach. So we stop that.

And then there is saffron. Saffron is a cure. If you have a lash and get an accident, you drink saffron to get rid of the clot. When you have a baby, you drink saffron. Sometimes, you cook the saffron in a little butter. You grate it, you cook it, its not runny and you make like a poultice or like a paste and you put it on the wound and you tie it. It will get rid of the clot underneath the skin. When you have a baby, saffron is a must, you must drink saffron.

## Midwifery and Postpartum

New mothers should know that saffron is a must. When you have a baby, drink a little saffron to get rid of all the little blood clots.

Then there is the hog plum bush. After you have the baby you would sit over a basin with hog plum bush. You boil it and bend over it and let it steam you inside and give you a good cleanse.

Keep ya foot warm when you have a baby. Wear socks or something, don't come outside barefeet because the cold will come through your foot and get into your body and get into your bones. Your body is open when you have a baby so all these things will get into you. And then when you nurse the baby you would pass it onto the baby.

And after you have a baby you can wash off or steam but you cannot bathe from your head to your foot. You had to wait 6 days and you had all these rituals and all this bush you had to get. And put it in the water and boil the bush in the water. Mash up some sweet broom [*Scoparia dulcis*] and hog plum bush [*Spondias mombin*] in the water and you bathe yourself for a cleansing. That was a cleansing for the body.

## Massages

When say like you fall or you play sports and it was hard or you jump down from somewhere and say oh gosh my belly hurting me. And you have a little diarrhea or upset stomach and you say ok leh we carry you by the neighbor to rub nara. So we take you to the neighbor and they feel your belly and they feel and they feel and they say ok you have nara. There is a lump here and your navel is beating too hard. THUMP THUMP THUMP! When its supposed to be a little easier doop doop doop. Its beating to hard you so you have a good nara! And they rub you down from your chest right down to your navel. And then they pull up from your private parts up towards your navel. They rub like that and then they rub on both sides. And then they turn you over and take the top of the hand and push your butt up up so the nara will go back in place.

INTERVIEWS AND BOTANICAL MUSINGS

Most of the rubbing was done with the coconut oil. The coconut oil had healing powers and that was available too. I learned from my mom and she learned from her mom. And I learn it too because when I had the nara and people rubbed me I would pay attention to what they are doing. Nara is like a muscle that you get a bump on the muscle. Like a tight muscle or a muscle out of place. And you have to rub that.

Jharay is another issue that is bad eye. Say your daughter is nice and pretty and she look good and the neighbor watching you with a bad eye, a cut eye. And then the child get sick. The child have a fever or the child have a runny nose and the next neighbor say I see the neighbor watching your child! She give the child maljo. She give the child maljo. Carry the child to get jharay. So there was always an elderly man or elderly woman in the village. Most times they are kind of holy people like pundit or a man who go to church all the time or woman who is always in the temple. And they say ok you go say good evening neighbor, I come to get the child jharay.

And they will chant a prayer but you do not hear exactly what they are saying. It's a secret prayer and sometimes they will take a little broom, one cocoyea broom, and touch the child easy on the shoulder and pray and pray and pray. But they don't let you hear what they are saying because I suppose the Hindu priest pundit have a different chant and the Muslim have a different chant. And I swear that the child feel good because the child feel good. Because that happened to us and my father took us to get jharay and we went and they prayed and they touched and sometimes they blow you like this. They blow away the evil eye from you and the child feel good. I know it because I take my small sister and my small brother and the child feel good and the child feel well.

Nowadays I don't know who you can go to because nowadays everyone believes in the pharmacy. If you sick, you go to the doctor, you go to the pharmacy.

CARIBBEAN HERBALISM

## Protection

Sometimes people would put a sticker on the child head to ward off the evil. They say that's the third eye to ward off the evil. Sometimes people put a sack with a little hing [asafoetida] in a little blue sack and they put it in the clothes where no one can see it to keep off the evil eye. You take a blue bottle and put it in the garden to ward off the evil eye. Blue always ward off the evil eye.

# THE DOSE MAKES THE POISON: ON CASTOR OIL AND SNAKE OIL

*This essay was originally published on Substack and edited for this book.*

"All things are poison, and nothing is without poison; the dosage alone makes it so a thing is not a poison." This old adage is usually attributed to Paracelsus in the early 1500s but has been found embodied in traditional medicine ways around the world from time immemorial. Traditional medicine has always been a complex dance with life and death, poison and healing potions. The medicine maker and communities held the knowledge of which plant killed and which one healed. Not only which plant, but which parts of plants and dosages create therapeutic effects versus unintended side effects.

A case study of the dose making the poison is castor bean (*Ricinus communis*, family Euphorbiaceae). I recently saw a large, robust, and shiny castor plant growing in a schoolyard here in Trinidad, and the principal asked if it was safe. As I smiled fondly at the plant, which is a deep source of inspiration for me, I had to let her know that although it is beautiful, the seeds contain a compound called ricin that in its concentrated version can kill a grown man over the course of two to four long, excruciating days. Just five to ten micrograms of pure ricin

INTERVIEWS AND BOTANICAL MUSINGS

per kilogram of body weight can be lethal. It inhibits protein synthesis, thereby killing cells permanently. On another note, this action of cell death is currently being explored in cancer research. This beautiful, enticing plant, which makes the beloved castor oil that many of us know and that is used in hundreds of traditional remedies around the world, can also kill you.

I personally have grown this plant for ten years, and I have saved its seeds for cultural and medicinal value. So, on the other hand, I can tell people about how the heated leaves have calmed pains and reduced inflammation in body parts. Or how the castor oil is extracted from the fatty seeds, using a process that deactivates the toxic ricin. I can talk about how castors are used for everything from biodiesel to bioterrorism to hair products to birth induction. It has a purgative nature that many Caribbean children will tell you

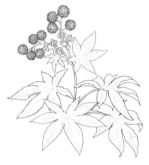

Castor

cleans you out real good and is given when people have colds or just as a seasonal cleanse.

This purgative effect is due to ricinoleic acid, which is the main fatty acid in castor oil. It binds to receptors on smooth muscle cells, which causes the intestinal muscles to contract and push contents through the system. Because you have smooth muscles all around your body, castor oil ingested in large doses can also cause contractions of the uterus, esophagus, and intestines. I have only used castor oil externally in salves and warm compresses. It really helps with wound healing and inflammation.

In Trinidad, many mothers are advised to drink castor oil nine days after giving birth to cleanse the womb, or even right before labor to help induce contractions. I cannot attest to the effects of this, however, because although I know it can work, I also recognize that the method of action is not the easiest on the whole body. There is a thin line between doing the job and overdoing the job, which would entail spending a whole day on the toilet!

So, as you can see, the dose or the method of ingestion makes the poison for castor bean and many other plants. Often, the most healing plants can also have the most toxicity, and that fascinates me. This is why it is important to learn about traditional uses and dosing of plants.

> [In the Border Cave in South Africa,] traces of wax containing ricinoleic and ricinelaidic acids were found on a thin wooden stick, which was suggested to be a poison applicator, dating back to about 24,000 years ago. The castor seeds and other parts of the castor plant were certainly utilized in ancient Egypt for pharmacological purposes. In the Ebers Papyrus, an Egyptian medical treatise dating back to before 1500 BCE, an entire chapter is dedicated to the castor bean that is indicated as an abortifacient, a laxative, a remedy for abscessual illness, baldness, and so on. In the Hearst Papyrus, written approximately in the same period, various castor plant parts are included as ingredients in some prescriptions for internal use, with the aim of expelling fluid accumulation or promoting diuresis, as well as for external use as poultices for bandaging. Ancient Egyptians knew the toxicity of castor bean and the use of seed pulp, included in drug preparations for oral ingestion, was recommended only in small amounts.[47]

Another toxic and healing plant genus that has come into my purview is the *Aristolochia* genus. Two members of that genus are named mat root (*Aristolochia rugosa*, family Aristolochiaceae) and tref root (*Aristolochia trilobata*), and they are well known as snakebite remedies and for their use in strong tonics for colds. Aristolochic acid, contained in *Aristolochia* plants, produces an increase in immune response, and it

---

47    L. Polito et al., "Ricin: An Ancient Story for a Timeless Plant Toxin," *Toxins* 11, no. 6 (2019): 324, doi: 10.3390/toxins11060324.

also inhibits the lytic activity (viral reproduction) of snake poison in the wound. In James Duke's book *Herb-a-Day*, he writes about how he would treat a snake bite in the wild:

> Rather fearful of proteolytic enzymes introduced into the wound, I might drink fig, papaya, or pineapple juice. We can assume that some of the birthworts (*Aristolochia*) around Explorama, like Virginia snakeroot back home, contain aristolochic acid which is said to inactivate snake venom. (But it is definitely a compound with which not to toy.)

At the same time as it can heal a snakebite, aristolochic acid in high doses acts as a nephrotoxin and carcinogen with very delayed effects. In the early 1990s, around 100 Belgian women started showing symptoms of rapidly progressing kidney failure that led to dialysis and kidney transplants. Investigators found that all of the women were taking the same weight loss supplement that had *Aristolochia fangchi*, an herb with medicinal effects used in traditional Chinese medicine. There is also a chronic kidney condition called Balkan endemic nephropathy. This is also seen in another Balkan region where the harvesting and milling of wheat involved the *Aristolochia clematitis* seeds being inevitably mixed with the wheat grains.[48]

In Trinidad, there is a low risk of our native *Aristolochia* species being mixed in our food supplies accidentally for slow poisoning. Or of you being one of the 5 percent of the population who suffer from a predisposition to kidney issues after prolonged exposure to aristolochic acid, according to an article in the *American Journal of Physiology: Renal Physiology*.[49]

---

48   A. P. Grollman and D. M. Marcus, "Global Hazards of Herbal Remedies: Lessons from *Aristolochia*," *EMBO Reports* 17, no. 5 (April 25, 2016): 619–25, doi: 10.15252/embr.201642375.

49   T. A. Rosenquist, "Genetic Loci That Affect Aristolochic Acid–Induced Nephrotoxicity in the Mouse," *AJP Renal Physiology* 300, no. 6 (June 1, 2011): F1360–67, doi: 10.1152/ajprenal.00716.2010.

Ethnobotanist Francis Morean of Trinidad and Tobago has countless articles and videos on his Facebook page about the uses of *Aristolochia* species in Trinidad (especially mat root and tref root). He often speaks to the potency of this herb for insulin regulation and the benefits of that on diabetes and PCOS patients. In addition to these uses, he has extensive experience and research on its use for snakebites and scorpion stings as well as its growing patterns. He also speaks to the fact that these herbs should only be taken with caution regarding dosage.

There are real risks and real benefits to the use of traditional herbs. They can be potent builders and destroyers of your body systems, and the action of phytochemicals in your body often mirrors the action in the plant where they were produced. For example, nicotine, coumarin, morphine, aristolochic acid, and ricin are all toxic compounds produced by plants as mechanisms to attract or repel organisms. And those same compounds have varying effects on the human body, from poison to pain relief to lifesaving. This is why I urge people to do research, build relationships with the plants they intend to use for healing, and, especially, learn from a skilled practitioner!

INTERVIEWS AND BOTANICAL MUSINGS

# APPENDIX A

# GLOSSARY OF TERMS

**alkaloids:** Nitrogen-containing compounds found in plants. They have a wide range of biological effects, such as pain relief, antibacterial activity, and immune system modulation. A well-known alkaloid is caffeine. Some alkaloids can be toxic, such as those found in deadly nightshade species.

**analgesic:** Compounds that reduce pain perception.

**antioxidants:** Compounds that reduce and reverse cellular stress and damage.

**astringent:** A property of a substance that makes it drying and tightening to tissues. Think of when you eat something sour.

**essential oil:** The natural oil contained in a plant that can be obtained through distillation. It is hyperconcentrated.

**liniment:** An herbal preparation that is meant for external use, to rub on skin.

**mucilage:** A polysaccharide compound that confers moistening and a viscous quality to mucous membranes. It protects and coats them. Mucilages act on tissues of the respiratory, gastrointestinal, and reproductive systems. Okra "slime" is an example of a mucilage.

**poultice:** A chewed, pounded, or blended herb that is placed on an affected area of skin.

**saponin:** A compound that makes things suds up or be soapy. Saponins are useful in shampoos and soaps and have many medicinal benefits.

**tannin:** A type of astringent that causes the dry feeling in your mouth when you drink certain bush teas or beverages like red wine.

**terpenes:** Aromatic compounds found in plants that are responsible for their fragrance. Many terpenes are bioactive.

# APPENDIX B

# COMMON AILMENTS AND ASSOCIATED HERBS

The following common conditions are traditionally treated with the herbs mentioned here and elsewhere in this book. This is solely for general information. If you want to treat yourself, you will need to reach out to a medical practitioner or an experienced herbalist to discuss dosage and plant parts to be used.

✿ **Anemia:** St. John's bush, railway daisy

✿ **Antidote:** mat root

✿ **Anti-inflammatory:** turmeric, railway daisy

✿ **Asthma:** carpenter grass, bois canot, malomay, genipa fruit, shark-liver oil

✿ **Blood pressure:** soursop, sorrel, guinea hen weed

✿ **Blood purification:** turmeric, aloes, guinea hen weed, zebapique, noni

✿ **Boils:** leaf of life, papaya

✿ **Bronchitis:** kooze mahoe, Congo lala

✿ **Colds:** seriyo, Spanish thyme, blue vervine, lime

- ❀ **Conjunctivitis:** ukee ukee, plantain
- ❀ **Constipation:** wild senna, castor oil
- ❀ **Cooling:** jigger bush, ditay payee, cerasee, lani bois
- ❀ **Coughs:** shandilay, bois canot
- ❀ **Cuts and wounds:** jigger bush, railway daisy, plantain, leaf of life
- ❀ **Diabetes:** mango leaf, neem, roucou, soursop, guinea hen weed
- ❀ **Dizziness:** soursop (crush leaves and smell)
- ❀ **Eczema:** cerasee, neem, wild senna, soapvine, St. John's bush
- ❀ **Epilepsy:** chadon beni
- ❀ **Fever:** Spanish thyme, fever grass
- ❀ **Fungal infections:** neem, coconut oil, cerasee, wild senna
- ❀ **Galactagogue:** blue vervine
- ❀ **Gastrointestinal issues:** papaya, Santa Maria, kooze mahoe, guava
- ❀ **Insomnia:** passionflower, barbadine, soursop, blue vervine
- ❀ **Kidney issues:** kooze mahoe, seed under leaf, purslane, ti-Marie
- ❀ **Low energy:** obi seed, cocoa
- ❀ **Menstrual issues:** monkey bone, cerasee, ginger, okra, sorrel
- ❀ **Mucilaginous:** okra, bois canot, aloe
- ❀ **Parasites:** barbadine, neem, cotton leaves
- ❀ **Purgative:** wild senna, castor oil, seriyo, aloe
- ❀ **Shampoo:** ratchette, bois canot, soap vine
- ❀ **Sinus issues:** guinea hen weed, railway daisy
- ❀ **Snakebite or scorpion sting:** mat root
- ❀ **Tooth pain:** guinea hen weed, lani bois, neem
- ❀ **Warming:** cinnamon, nutmeg

COMMON AILMENTS AND ASSOCIATED HERBS

## APPENDIX C

# RESEARCH TIPS

To build a deeper understanding of how a plant works, here are some research tips:

- ❁ Get familiar with the iNaturalist app. The photo identification feature is not always accurate, but you can use known and verified photos of plants to cross-reference with a specimen you are trying to identify. Upload photos and wait for humans within the app to identify your plant, rather than relying on the "Guess what this is?" feature.

- ❁ Create a Google Drive folder to hold notes, pictures, research articles, and the like.

- ❁ Sign up for free or paid subscriptions on sites such as Scribd, ResearchGate, and Academia.edu.

- ❁ Searching plants under their Latin name rather than their common name will yield more results on an internet search. For example, type "Latin name of carpenter grass" and then go to the Images tab and find the plant that looks like what you are searching for. Take note of the Latin name and then search for "traditional uses/ethnobotany of/medicinal uses of Justicia pectoralis." If I search for "Justicia pectoralis + Guyana," a different common name would be shown (toyeu or toyo).

❀ You will think you will remember where you found a piece of information, but you won't. So be sure to bookmark pages or take notes listing the sites or books you are using.

❀ Visit your local horticultural societies, foraging groups, botanical gardens, libraries, or herbaria for more resources on plant identification.

❀ Search the Latin name of a plant + toxicity or poisonous look-alikes if you want to double-check the safety of an herb you want to use or that you recently foraged.

❀ Remember that there is a lot of false information on the internet and viral memes with strong claims. Do your own diligence to not fall for clickbait or confirmation bias. I recommend going to libraries to see and cite real books, research articles, or firsthand experience. Local libraries often have great herbal and botanical resource books.

❀ Interview people in your community about herbs. You get bonus points if they are elders!

❀ Search in different languages using the plant name and use Google Translate. Sometimes an herb may be popular in Brazil, for example, and a lot of good recipes or articles may be in Portuguese and not show up in your internet search.

❀ If you are unsure of how toxic a plant is, I recommend searching Latin name + toxicity or precautions. You can also search for poisonous look-alikes, if you are uncertain of an identification.

RESEARCH TIPS

# ACKNOWLEDGMENTS

I would like to preface this work by giving all thanks to the Most High, Yahweh, for providing this platform and this channel to share this knowledge. I have been granted so much goodness and mercy through this journey, and at the end and the beginning of the day, I give thanks!

I have been blessed with many mentors and guides over the years who have inspired me, taught me, and guided my studies, and I would be remiss if I did not acknowledge them. I would like to thank my husband for his steadfast love, guidance, and support; my parents and sister for always supporting my dreams; my Grandmother May for being a prayer warrior and the first person to introduce me to bush medicine; my mother-in-law, Gloria Parris, for sharing so much of her herbal knowledge with me; Francis Morean for sharing extensive knowledge of ethnobotany and for allowing me to learn from him and use his interviews in this book; Henriette den Ouden for my first botanical immersion with tulsi (holy basil); the late James Duke for his teachings and his Green Pharmacy legacy; the staff and curator from the National Herbarium of Trinidad and Tobago for their research support and encouragement; every elder and bush person who has shared knowledge with me over the years; and my daughter for being a catalyst for me to document this knowledge for her and future generations!

This book would not have been possible without generations of knowledge being passed down and practiced. It would not have happened without God's guidance to the right places and teachers and environments to foster my learning. For these things, and these plants, I am grateful.

# ABOUT THE AUTHOR

Aleya Fraser is a land steward and ethnobotanist with a strong lineage of land-based people. She has spent the last 12 years managing and founding farms and deepening her herbal knowledge through communing with elders, practice, and scientific research. Aleya uses her bachelor's degree in physiology and neurobiology as well as the ancestral wisdom in her fingertips to guide her studies and research interests. She blends her upbringing in Maryland with a strong focus on Trinidadian roots in her writings. She is considered a pollinator of people and weaver of landscapes.

Aleya also managed and cofounded farms in Baltimore City, on the Eastern Shore of Maryland, in Northwest Virginia, and now, in her ancestral lands of Trinidad and Tobago, where she lives with her husband and daughter. She can be found on social media at @naturaleya or naturaleya.substack.com or caribbeanherbalism.com.